No Gallbladder

Diet Cookbook

300+ Days of Delicious Recipes to Support Your Healthy Diet and Body Post-Gallbladder Removal

Includes a 30-Day Meal Plan with Organic Ingredients and Supplements for Effective Bile Production and Digestion Support for Beginners

Barbara Flowers

Table of Contents

Introduction

Welcome to Your New Journey

Welcome to "No Gallbladder Diet Cookbook: 300+ Days of Delicious Recipes to Support Your Healthy Diet and Body Post-Gallbladder Removal." This cookbook is designed specifically for those who have undergone gallbladder removal and are looking for delicious, healthy, and easy-to-prepare meals to support their digestive health and overall well-being.

Life after gallbladder surgery can present unique dietary challenges. Without a gallbladder, your body needs a bit of extra help to digest fats and absorb nutrients efficiently. This book provides a comprehensive 30-day meal plan featuring recipes made with organic ingredients and supplements to aid bile production and digestion. Our goal is to make your transition to a new diet as smooth and enjoyable as possible.

In the following pages, you will find a carefully curated collection of recipes that cater to your nutritional needs while offering a variety of flavors and textures. From hearty breakfasts to satisfying lunches, dinners, snacks, and desserts, each recipe has been crafted with your health in mind. Let's embark on this journey together, embracing a new lifestyle that nourishes your body and delights your taste buds.

Welcome to your new culinary adventure!

How This Cookbook Can Help You

This cookbook is your guide to navigating the dietary changes that come with life after gallbladder removal. We understand that adjusting to a new way of eating can feel overwhelming, especially when trying to balance flavor, nutrition, and digestibility. That's why we've designed this book to help you every step of the way.

What You'll Find Inside:

- **A 30-Day Meal Plan:** A structured meal plan specifically designed to support your digestive health and ease your transition to a new diet. Each day includes five delicious recipes for breakfast, lunch, dinner, snacks, and desserts that are easy to prepare and packed with nutrients.
- **Simple, Tasty Recipes:** Our recipes focus on using whole, natural ingredients that are gentle on your digestive system while still being delicious. You'll find a variety of meals that cater to different tastes and preferences, ensuring you never get bored of your new diet.
- **Digestive Health Support:** Each recipe is crafted to promote effective digestion and support bile production, which is crucial after gallbladder removal. We've included tips and suggestions to help you understand which foods are most beneficial for your unique needs.
- **Practical Guidance:** Beyond recipes, this book offers practical tips for meal preparation, kitchen organization, and smart shopping, all tailored to help you maintain your new diet with ease. You'll learn how to plan your meals ahead, make the most of your ingredients, and avoid common pitfalls.

By following the guidance in this cookbook, you'll be equipped with the knowledge and tools you need to thrive on a gallbladder-friendly diet. Our goal is to empower you to take charge of your health with confidence and enjoy a variety of foods that support your body's new needs.

With this cookbook, you can look forward to a journey of recovery filled with flavor, nutrition, and satisfaction. Let's get started!

1   Part 1: Getting Started

Overview of the 30-Day Meal Plan

The 30-Day Meal Plan is designed to help you transition smoothly to a gallbladder-friendly diet while enjoying a variety of delicious and nutritious meals. Each day includes five meals: breakfast, lunch, dinner, snacks, and dessert. The meal plan focuses on:

- **Balanced Nutrition:** Each meal is carefully crafted to provide a balance of macronutrients (proteins, carbohydrates, and fats) that are easy to digest and supportive of your body's needs post-gallbladder removal.
- **Simple, Digestible Ingredients:** The recipes prioritize ingredients that are gentle on the digestive system, helping to minimize discomfort and promote effective digestion.

- **Variety and Flavor:** To keep your meals exciting, the plan includes a diverse range of flavors, textures, and cuisines, ensuring you enjoy your food while sticking to your dietary needs.
- **Ease of Preparation:** All meals are designed to be simple and quick to prepare, making it easy for you to follow the plan without spending hours in the kitchen.

By following this 30-Day Meal Plan, you will establish healthy eating habits, learn how to prepare gallbladder-friendly meals, and support your overall well-being. This plan serves as a foundation for maintaining a healthy diet long-term. Let's get started on this path to better health with confidence and delicious meals!

2   Preparing Your Kitchen for Success

A well-prepared kitchen is key to successfully following a new diet, especially after gallbladder removal. Setting up your kitchen with the right tools, ingredients, and organization can make meal preparation smoother and more enjoyable. Here are some essential steps to help you get started:

1. Stock Up on Gallbladder-Friendly Staples

Ensure your pantry and fridge are filled with ingredients that support your new diet. Focus on whole, unprocessed foods that are easy to digest and promote healthy bile production. Key items to have on hand include:

- Fresh fruits and vegetables (like leafy greens, carrots, and apples)
- Lean proteins (such as chicken, turkey, fish, and tofu)
- Whole grains (like quinoa, brown rice, and oats)
- Healthy fats (including olive oil, avocados, and nuts)
- Low-fat dairy or dairy alternatives (like almond milk or Greek yogurt)

2. Organize Your Kitchen for Efficiency

Make your kitchen a stress-free environment by organizing it for easy access to your cooking essentials. Keep frequently used items like cutting boards, knives, and measuring cups within reach. Arrange your pantry so that healthier options are at the front and visible.

3. Invest in Essential Kitchen Tools

Having the right kitchen tools can make a big difference in meal preparation. Consider investing in these essential items:

- Non-stick pans and pots for low-fat cooking
- A food processor or blender for smoothies and purees
- Sharp knives for easy chopping and slicing
- Airtight containers for storing pre-prepped ingredients and leftovers

4. Prepare Ingredients Ahead of Time

To save time and reduce stress, consider prepping ingredients ahead of time. Wash and chop vegetables, cook grains, and portion out snacks in advance. This makes it easier to throw together a quick meal or snack when you're pressed for time or energy.

5. Plan Your Meals and Grocery Shopping

Plan your meals for the week based on the 30-Day Meal Plan. Create a shopping list that includes all the ingredients you'll need, which helps avoid unnecessary purchases and ensures you always have the right foods on hand. This will make it easier to stick to your diet and avoid temptations.

By preparing your kitchen and organizing your space, you set yourself up for success in following the 30-Day Meal Plan and maintaining a healthy, gallbladder-friendly diet. A little preparation goes a long way in ensuring your new dietary habits are sustainable and enjoyable. Let's get cooking!

3 Part 2: The 30-Day Meal Plan
Week 1: Easing Into Your New Diet

Day 1

Breakfast: Oatmeal with Fresh Berries and Honey

Ingredients:

- 1 cup rolled oats
- 2 cups water or almond milk
- 1/2 cup fresh berries (such as blueberries, strawberries, or raspberries)
- 1 tablespoon honey
- 1/4 teaspoon cinnamon (optional)
- A pinch of salt

Instructions:

1. **Prepare the Oats:** In a medium saucepan, bring the water or almond milk to a boil. Add a pinch of salt and the rolled oats, stirring occasionally. Reduce the heat to low and let simmer for about 5 minutes, or until the oats are tender and the liquid is absorbed.

2. **Add Flavor:** Stir in the cinnamon, if using, to add a hint of spice and warmth to your oatmeal.

3. **Top with Berries and Honey:** Transfer the oatmeal to a bowl. Top with fresh berries of your choice for a burst of natural sweetness and color. Drizzle with honey for added flavor and sweetness.

Lunch: Grilled Chicken Salad with Light Vinaigrette

Ingredients:

- 1 boneless, skinless chicken breast
- 1 tablespoon olive oil
- Salt and pepper to taste
- 4 cups mixed salad greens (such as romaine, spinach, and arugula)
- 1/2 cup cherry tomatoes, halved

For the Light Vinaigrette:

- 2 tablespoons olive oil
- 1 tablespoon apple cider vinegar or lemon juice
- 1 teaspoon Dijon mustard

- 1/4 cucumber, sliced
- 1/4 red onion, thinly sliced
- 1/4 cup shredded carrots
- 1/4 avocado, sliced
- 2 tablespoons feta cheese (optional)

- 1 teaspoon honey
- Salt and pepper to taste

Instructions:

1. **Prepare the Chicken:**
   o Preheat a grill or grill pan over medium-high heat.
   o Brush the chicken breast with olive oil and season with salt and pepper.
   o Grill the chicken for about 6-7 minutes on each side or until fully cooked and the internal temperature reaches 165°F (75°C). Remove from the grill and let rest for a few minutes before slicing.

2. **Prepare the Salad:**
   o While the chicken is grilling, prepare the salad ingredients. In a large bowl, combine the mixed salad greens, cherry tomatoes, cucumber, red onion, shredded carrots, and avocado slices.

3. **Make the Vinaigrette:**
   o In a small bowl or jar, whisk together the olive oil, apple cider vinegar or lemon juice, Dijon mustard, honey, salt, and pepper until well combined. Adjust seasoning to taste.

4. **Assemble the Salad:**
   o Slice the grilled chicken breast into thin strips and add it to the salad. Drizzle the light vinaigrette over the salad and toss gently to coat all ingredients evenly.

Dinner: Baked Salmon with Steamed Vegetables

Ingredients:

- 2 salmon fillets (about 4-6 ounces each)
- 1 tablespoon olive oil
- 1 lemon (half sliced, half for juice)
- 2 cloves garlic, minced

- 1 teaspoon fresh dill or parsley, chopped (optional)
- Salt and pepper to taste
- 1 cup broccoli florets
- 1 cup carrots, sliced
- 1 cup zucchini, sliced

Instructions:

1. **Preheat the Oven:**
   - Preheat your oven to 375°F (190°C).
2. **Prepare the Salmon:**
   - Place the salmon fillets on a baking sheet lined with parchment paper or lightly greased with olive oil.
   - Drizzle the fillets with olive oil and lemon juice. Season with minced garlic, salt, and pepper. Add a few lemon slices on top of the salmon for extra flavor. Sprinkle with fresh dill or parsley if using.
3. **Bake the Salmon:**
   - Bake in the preheated oven for 12-15 minutes, or until the salmon is cooked through and flakes easily with a fork. Cooking time may vary depending on the thickness of the fillets.
4. **Prepare the Vegetables:**
   - While the salmon is baking, prepare the vegetables. In a steamer basket over boiling water, add the broccoli, carrots, and zucchini. Cover and steam for about 5-7 minutes or until the vegetables are tender but still crisp.

Snack: Sliced Apples with Almond Butter

Ingredients:

- 1 medium apple (such as Fuji, Honeycrisp, or Gala)
- 2 tablespoons almond butter (unsweetened and smooth)
- A sprinkle of cinnamon (optional)

Instructions:

1. **Prepare the Apple:**
   - Wash the apple thoroughly under running water. Cut the apple into thin slices, discarding the core and seeds.
2. **Serve with Almond Butter:**
   - Arrange the apple slices on a plate. Serve with a small bowl or spoonful of almond butter on the side for dipping.
3. **Add a Flavor Boost (Optional):**
   - Sprinkle a light dusting of cinnamon over the apple slices for an added hint of warmth and flavor.

Dessert: Chia Seed Pudding with Coconut Milk

Ingredients:

- 1/4 cup chia seeds
- 1 cup unsweetened coconut milk (from a carton, not canned)
- 1 tablespoon maple syrup or honey
- 1/2 teaspoon vanilla extract
- Fresh fruit for topping (such as berries, mango, or kiwi)
- A sprinkle of shredded coconut (optional)

Instructions:

1. **Mix the Ingredients:**
   - In a bowl or a jar, combine the chia seeds, coconut milk, maple syrup (or honey), and vanilla extract. Stir well to ensure that the chia seeds are evenly distributed and not clumping together.
2. **Refrigerate the Pudding:**
   - Cover the bowl or jar and refrigerate for at least 2 hours, or preferably overnight. The chia seeds will absorb

the coconut milk and expand, creating a pudding-like consistency.

3. **Stir and Check Consistency:**
   - After the pudding has set, stir it well to ensure an even texture. If the pudding is too thick for your liking, you can add a bit more coconut milk and stir again.

4. **Serve with Toppings:**
   - Spoon the chia seed pudding into serving bowls or glasses. Top with fresh fruit of your choice, such as berries, diced mango, or kiwi. For added texture and flavor, sprinkle a little shredded coconut on top.

Day 2

Breakfast: Green Smoothie with Spinach, Banana, and Avocado

Ingredients:

- 1 cup fresh spinach leaves
- 1 ripe banana
- 1/2 ripe avocado
- 1 cup unsweetened almond milk (or your preferred dairy-free milk)
- 1 tablespoon chia seeds (optional)
- 1 teaspoon honey or maple syrup (optional, for added sweetness)
- Ice cubes (optional, for a colder smoothie)

Instructions:

1. **Prepare the Ingredients:**
   - Wash the spinach leaves thoroughly under running water.
   - Peel the banana and avocado. Slice the banana and scoop out the avocado flesh.
2. **Blend the Smoothie:**
   - In a blender, combine the spinach, banana, avocado, almond milk, and chia seeds (if using).
   - Blend on high until the mixture is smooth and creamy. If you prefer a colder smoothie, add a few ice cubes and blend again until smooth.
3. **Sweeten to Taste:**
   - Taste the smoothie. If you prefer a sweeter flavor, add a teaspoon of honey or maple syrup and blend briefly to combine.

Lunch: Quinoa Salad with Cucumber, Tomatoes, and Feta

Ingredients:

- 1 cup quinoa, rinsed
- 2 cups water
- 1 cup cucumber, diced
- 1 cup cherry tomatoes, halved
- 1/4 cup red onion, finely chopped
- 1/4 cup crumbled feta cheese
- 2 tablespoons fresh parsley, chopped
- 2 tablespoons olive oil
- 1 tablespoon lemon juice
- Salt and pepper to taste

Instructions:

1. **Cook the Quinoa:**
   - In a medium saucepan, bring 2 cups of water to a boil. Add the rinsed quinoa and reduce the heat to low. Cover and simmer for about 15 minutes, or until the quinoa is tender and the water is absorbed. Remove from heat and let it cool to room temperature.
2. **Prepare the Vegetables:**
   - While the quinoa is cooking, prepare the vegetables. Dice the cucumber, halve the cherry tomatoes, and finely chop the red onion. Chop the fresh parsley as well.
3. **Combine Ingredients:**
   - In a large mixing bowl, combine the cooked and cooled quinoa, cucumber, cherry tomatoes, red onion, and parsley. Add the crumbled feta cheese.
4. **Make the Dressing:**
   - In a small bowl, whisk together the olive oil, lemon juice, salt, and pepper until well combined.
5. **Dress the Salad:**
   - Pour the dressing over the quinoa and vegetable mixture. Toss gently to ensure everything is evenly coated with the dressing

Dinner: Chicken and Vegetable Stir-Fry

Ingredients:

- 1-pound boneless, skinless chicken breast, sliced into thin strips
- 2 tablespoons olive oil or sesame oil
- 2 cloves garlic, minced
- 1 teaspoon fresh ginger, minced
- 1 red bell pepper, sliced
- 1 cup broccoli florets
- 1 cup snap peas
- 1 medium carrot, thinly sliced
- 1 small zucchini, sliced
- 2 tablespoons low-sodium soy sauce or tamari (gluten-free option)
- 1 tablespoon honey or maple syrup
- 1 tablespoon rice vinegar
- 1 teaspoon cornstarch (optional, for thickening)
- 1/4 cup water
- 2 tablespoons green onions, chopped (optional, for garnish)
- Cooked brown rice or quinoa, for serving

Instructions:

1. **Prepare the Sauce:**
   - In a small bowl, whisk together the low-sodium soy sauce (or tamari), honey or maple syrup, rice vinegar, and cornstarch (if using). Add the water and mix until smooth. Set aside.
2. **Cook the Chicken:**
   - Heat 1 tablespoon of olive oil or sesame oil in a large skillet or wok over medium-high heat. Add the sliced chicken breast and cook until it is browned and fully cooked through, about 5-7 minutes. Remove the chicken from the skillet and set aside.
3. **Stir-Fry the Vegetables:**
   - In the same skillet, add the remaining tablespoon of oil. Add the minced garlic and ginger and sauté for about 30 seconds until fragrant.
   - Add the sliced red bell pepper, broccoli florets, snap peas, carrot, and zucchini. Stir-fry the vegetables for about 5-7 minutes, or until they are tender-crisp.
4. **Combine Chicken and Sauce:**
   - Return the cooked chicken to the skillet with the vegetables. Pour the prepared sauce over the chicken and vegetables. Stir well to coat everything evenly.
5. **Thicken the Sauce (Optional):**

- o If you used cornstarch in the sauce, cook for an additional 1-2 minutes until the sauce has thickened and everything is heated through.
6. **Serve and Garnish:**

- o Serve the chicken and vegetable stir-fry over cooked brown rice or quinoa. Garnish with chopped green onions if desired.

Snack: Carrot Sticks with Hummus

Ingredients:

- 2 large carrots, peeled and cut into sticks
-

- 1/2 cup hummus (store-bought or homemade)

Optional Hummus Ingredients (for homemade):

- 1 can (15 ounces) chickpeas, drained and rinsed
- 2 tablespoons tahini
- 2 tablespoons olive oil
- 1-2 tablespoons lemon juice
- 1 garlic clove, minced

- 1/2 teaspoon ground cumin
- Salt to taste
- Water, as needed, for desired consistency

Instructions:

1. **Prepare the Carrot Sticks:**
   - o Peel the carrots and cut them into sticks, about 3-4 inches long and 1/4 inch thick. Set aside.
2. **Make the Hummus (if homemade):**
   - o In a food processor, combine the chickpeas, tahini, olive oil, lemon juice, minced garlic, cumin, and salt. Blend until smooth.
   - o If the hummus is too thick, add a tablespoon of water at a time until the desired consistency is reached. Adjust seasoning to taste.
3. **Serve the Snack:**
   - o Arrange the carrot sticks on a plate and serve with a side of hummus for dipping.

Dessert: Baked Pear with Cinnamon and Honey

Ingredients:

- 2 ripe pears, halved and cored
- 1 tablespoon honey
- 1/2 teaspoon ground cinnamon
- 1/4 teaspoon vanilla extract (optional)

- A handful of chopped nuts (such as walnuts or almonds, optional)
- Greek yogurt or a dollop of whipped cream (optional, for serving)

Instructions:

1. **Preheat the Oven:**
   - Preheat your oven to 350°F (175°C).
2. **Prepare the Pears:**
   - Cut the pears in half lengthwise and remove the core using a spoon or a melon baller. Arrange the pear halves in a baking dish, cut side up.
3. **Add Honey and Cinnamon:**
   - Drizzle the honey over the pears, making sure to cover each half evenly. Sprinkle the ground cinnamon over the top. Add a few drops of vanilla extract to each pear half, if using.
4. **Bake the Pears:**
   - Place the baking dish in the preheated oven and bake for 20-25 minutes, or until the pears are tender and golden brown. The baking time may vary depending on the ripeness of the pears.
5. **Optional Toppings:**
   - If desired, sprinkle chopped nuts over the pears during the last 5 minutes of baking for added crunch and flavor.

Day 3

Breakfast: Scrambled Eggs with Spinach and Mushrooms

Ingredients:

- 2 large eggs
- 1/4 cup fresh spinach leaves, chopped
- 1/4 cup mushrooms, sliced
- 1 tablespoon olive oil or butter
- 1 tablespoon milk or water (optional, for fluffier eggs)
- Salt and pepper to taste
- 1 tablespoon fresh chives or parsley, chopped (optional, for garnish)

Instructions:

1. **Prepare the Ingredients:**
   - Wash and chop the spinach leaves. Slice the mushrooms. Crack the eggs into a small bowl, add milk or water (if using), and whisk until well combined. Season with a pinch of salt and pepper.
2. **Cook the Vegetables:**
   - Heat a non-stick skillet over medium heat and add the olive oil or butter. Once hot, add the sliced mushrooms and sauté for 2-3 minutes, or until they start to soften.
3. **Add Spinach:**
   - Add the chopped spinach to the skillet with the mushrooms. Sauté for another 1-2 minutes until the spinach wilts.
4. **Scramble the Eggs:**

o   Pour the whisked eggs into the skillet with the vegetables. Let them sit undisturbed for a few seconds, then gently stir with a spatula, pushing the eggs from the edges toward the center as they cook.

5. **Cook to Desired Consistency:**
    o   Continue cooking the eggs, stirring occasionally, until they reach your desired level of doneness. Remove from heat while the eggs are still slightly soft, as they will continue to cook from residual heat.

6. **Serve and Garnish:**
    o   Transfer the scrambled eggs with spinach and mushrooms to a plate. Garnish with fresh chives or parsley if desired.

Lunch: Lentil Soup with Whole Grain Bread

Ingredients:

- 1 cup dried lentils (green or brown), rinsed and drained
- 1 tablespoon olive oil
- 1 medium onion, diced
- 2 cloves garlic, minced
- 2 carrots, diced
- 2 celery stalks, diced
- 1 medium tomato, diced (or 1/2 cup canned diced tomatoes)
- 1 teaspoon ground cumin
- 1/2 teaspoon ground turmeric
- 1/2 teaspoon paprika
- 4 cups low-sodium vegetable or chicken broth
- 1 bay leaf
- Salt and pepper to taste
- 2 tablespoons fresh parsley, chopped (optional, for garnish)
- 4 slices of whole grain bread

Instructions:

1. **Sauté the Vegetables:**
    o   In a large pot, heat the olive oil over medium heat. Add the diced onion, carrots, and celery, and sauté for about 5 minutes until the vegetables are softened.

2. **Add Garlic and Spices:**
    o   Add the minced garlic and cook for another 1-2 minutes until fragrant. Stir in the ground cumin, turmeric, and paprika, and cook for 30 seconds to release their flavors.

3. **Add Lentils and Tomatoes:**
    o   Add the rinsed lentils and diced tomatoes to the pot, stirring to combine with the vegetables and spices.

4. **Add Broth and Simmer:**
    o   Pour in the low-sodium vegetable or chicken broth and add the bay leaf. Bring the mixture to a boil, then reduce the heat to low and let it simmer for about 25-30 minutes, or until the lentils are tender.

5. **Season and Finish:**
    o   Once the lentils are cooked, remove the bay leaf. Season the soup with salt and pepper to taste. If the soup is too thick, you can add a bit more broth or water to reach your desired consistency.

6. **Serve the Soup:**
    o   Ladle the lentil soup into bowls and garnish with fresh parsley if desired.

7. **Serve with Whole Grain Bread:**
    o   Serve the soup with slices of whole grain bread on the side for dipping. You can lightly toast the bread for added texture.

Dinner: Grilled Shrimp with Brown Rice and Asparagus

Ingredients:

- 1-pound large shrimp, peeled and deveined
- 1 tablespoon olive oil
- 2 cloves garlic, minced
- 1 teaspoon lemon zest
- Juice of 1 lemon
- Salt and pepper to taste
- 1 cup brown rice
- 2 cups water or low-sodium chicken broth
- 1 bunch asparagus, trimmed
- 1 tablespoon olive oil (for asparagus)
- 1 tablespoon fresh parsley, chopped (optional, for garnish)
- Lemon wedges (optional, for serving)

Instructions:

1. **Prepare the Brown Rice:**
   - In a medium saucepan, bring 2 cups of water or low-sodium chicken broth to a boil. Add the brown rice, reduce heat to low, cover, and simmer for about 40-45 minutes, or until the rice is tender and the liquid is absorbed. Remove from heat and let sit, covered, for 5 minutes before fluffing with a fork.
2. **Marinate the Shrimp:**
   - In a bowl, combine the shrimp, olive oil, minced garlic, lemon zest, lemon juice, salt, and pepper. Toss to coat the shrimp evenly. Let the shrimp marinate for about 10-15 minutes while you prepare the asparagus.
3. **Prepare the Asparagus:**
   - Preheat a grill or grill pan over medium-high heat. Toss the trimmed asparagus with olive oil, salt, and pepper.
4. **Grill the Shrimp and Asparagus:**
   - Place the shrimp on skewers (if using a grill) or directly on the grill pan. Grill the shrimp for about 2-3 minutes per side, or until they are pink and opaque. Be careful not to overcook the shrimp.
   - At the same time, grill the asparagus, turning occasionally, for about 5-7 minutes, or until tender and slightly charred.
5. **Serve the Meal:**
   - Divide the brown rice among plates. Top with grilled shrimp and asparagus. Garnish with fresh parsley if desired.
6. **Optional Garnish:**
   - Serve with lemon wedges on the side for an extra squeeze of fresh lemon juice.

Snack: Greek Yogurt with Honey and Walnuts

Ingredients:

- 1 cup Greek yogurt (plain, unsweetened)
- 1 tablespoon honey
- 2 tablespoons walnuts, chopped
- A pinch of cinnamon (optional)

Instructions:

1. **Prepare the Yogurt:**
   - Scoop the Greek yogurt into a small bowl.

2. **Add Toppings:**
   - o Drizzle the honey over the yogurt. Sprinkle the chopped walnuts on top for a crunchy texture.

3. **Optional Flavor Boost:**
   - o For an extra hint of warmth and flavor, add a pinch of cinnamon on top.

Dessert: Fresh Fruit Salad with Mint

Ingredients:

- 1 cup strawberries, hulled and sliced
- 1 cup blueberries
- 1 cup pineapple, diced
- 1 kiwi, peeled and sliced
- 1 orange, peeled and segmented
- 1/2 cup grapes, halved
- 1 tablespoon fresh mint leaves, finely chopped
- 1 tablespoon honey or fresh lemon juice (optional, for added sweetness or a tangy kick)

Instructions:

1. **Prepare the Fruit:**
   - o Wash all the fruit thoroughly. Hull and slice the strawberries, dice the pineapple, peel and slice the kiwi, peel and segment the orange, and halve the grapes.
2. **Combine the Fruit:**
   - o In a large mixing bowl, combine the strawberries, blueberries, pineapple, kiwi, orange, and grapes.
3. **Add Mint and Optional Ingredients:**
   - o Sprinkle the finely chopped mint leaves over the fruit mixture. If desired, drizzle honey for added sweetness or a splash of fresh lemon juice for a tangy flavor.
4. **Toss and Chill:**
   - o Gently toss the fruit salad to combine all the ingredients evenly. Refrigerate for about 15-20 minutes to allow the flavors to meld and the fruit to chill slightly.

Day 4

Breakfast: Smoothie Bowl with Mixed Berries and Granola

Ingredients:

- 1 cup frozen mixed berries (such as strawberries, blueberries, raspberries, and blackberries)
- 1/2 ripe banana
- 1/2 cup unsweetened almond milk (or your preferred dairy-free milk)

- 1/2 cup plain Greek yogurt (or a dairy-free alternative)
- 1 tablespoon honey or maple syrup (optional, for added sweetness)

Toppings:

- 1/4 cup granola (choose a low-sugar variety)
- Fresh berries (such as sliced strawberries, blueberries, or raspberries)
- Sliced banana
- 1 tablespoon chia seeds or flaxseeds (optional)
- 1 tablespoon shredded coconut (optional)
- 1 tablespoon sliced almonds or other nuts (optional)

Instructions:

1. **Blend the Smoothie Base:**
   - In a blender, combine the frozen mixed berries, half a banana, unsweetened almond milk, Greek yogurt, and honey or maple syrup (if using). Blend until smooth and thick. If the mixture is too thick, you can add a little more almond milk to reach your desired consistency.
2. **Pour and Spread:**
   - Pour the smoothie mixture into a bowl. Use a spoon to spread it evenly to create a nice, smooth base.
3. **Add Toppings:**
   - Top the smoothie bowl with granola for crunch, fresh berries, and sliced banana for extra flavor and texture. Sprinkle chia seeds or flaxseeds, shredded coconut, and sliced almonds on top, if desired.

Lunch: Turkey and Avocado Wrap

Ingredients:

- 1 whole wheat or gluten-free tortilla
- 4-5 slices of roasted turkey breast (preferably low sodium)
- 1/2 ripe avocado, sliced
- 1/4 cup mixed greens (such as spinach, arugula, or lettuce)
- 1/4 cup cucumber, thinly sliced
- 1/4 cup tomato, thinly sliced
- 1 tablespoon hummus or Greek yogurt (optional, for added flavor)
- Salt and pepper to taste

Instructions:

1. **Prepare the Ingredients:**
   - Slice the avocado, cucumber, and tomato. Set aside all the ingredients for easy assembly.
2. **Lay Out the Tortilla:**
   - Place the whole wheat or gluten-free tortilla flat on a clean surface or plate.
3. **Add the Spread (Optional):**
   - If using hummus or Greek yogurt, spread it evenly over the tortilla to add flavor and help hold the ingredients together.
4. **Layer the Ingredients:**
   - Lay the roasted turkey slices on the tortilla. Add the avocado slices, mixed greens, cucumber, and tomato on top of the turkey. Season with a pinch of salt and pepper to taste.
5. **Roll the Wrap:**
   - Carefully roll the tortilla tightly, folding in the sides as you go to keep the ingredients inside. You can secure the wrap with a toothpick if needed.
6. **Slice and Serve:**
   - Slice the wrap in half diagonally for easy eating. Serve immediately.

Dinner: Zucchini Noodles with Tomato Basil Sauce

Ingredients:

- 2 medium zucchinis, spiralized into noodles (zoodles)
- 1 tablespoon olive oil
- 2 cloves garlic, minced
- 1 can (15 ounces) diced tomatoes; no salt added
- 1/2 teaspoon dried oregano
- 1/2 teaspoon dried basil
- Salt and pepper to taste
- 1/4 cup fresh basil leaves, chopped
- 1/4 cup grated Parmesan cheese (optional)
- Red pepper flakes (optional, for a bit of heat)

Instructions:

1. **Prepare the Zucchini Noodles:**
   - Using a spiralizer, turn the zucchinis into noodles (zoodles). If you don't have a spiralizer, you can use a vegetable peeler to create thin ribbons or julienne them by hand.

2. **Make the Tomato Basil Sauce:**
   - In a large skillet, heat the olive oil over medium heat. Add the minced garlic and sauté for about 1 minute until fragrant.
   - Add the diced tomatoes, dried oregano, and dried basil to the skillet. Stir well to combine. Bring the sauce to a simmer and let it cook for about 10-15 minutes, allowing the flavors to meld together. Season with salt and pepper to taste.

3. **Cook the Zucchini Noodles:**
   - In a separate skillet, add a small amount of olive oil and heat over medium heat. Add the zucchini noodles and sauté for about 2-3 minutes, just until they are tender but still slightly crisp. Be careful not to overcook the zoodles, as they can become mushy.

4. **Combine Noodles and Sauce:**
   - Add the cooked zucchini noodles to the skillet with the tomato basil sauce. Toss gently to coat the noodles evenly with the sauce.

5. **Serve and Garnish:**
   - Divide the zucchini noodles with tomato basil sauce among serving plates. Top with fresh basil leaves and a sprinkle of grated Parmesan cheese if desired. Add red pepper flakes for a bit of heat, if using.

Snack: Celery Sticks with Cottage Cheese

Ingredients:

- 2-3 celery stalks, cut into sticks
- 1/2 cup cottage cheese (low-fat or full fat, based on preference)
- A pinch of black pepper (optional, for seasoning)
- A sprinkle of paprika or chopped fresh herbs (such as parsley or chives) (optional, for garnish)

Instructions:

1. **Prepare the Celery Sticks:**
   - Wash the celery stalks thoroughly under running water. Cut each stalk into sticks, about 3-4 inches long.

2. **Serve the Cottage Cheese:**
   - o Spoon the cottage cheese into a small bowl. If desired, sprinkle with black

pepper, paprika, or fresh herbs for added flavor and a pop of color.

3. **Assemble the Snack:**
   - o Arrange the celery sticks on a plate alongside the cottage cheese.

Dessert: Dark Chocolate-Covered Strawberries

Ingredients:

- 1 cup fresh strawberries, washed and dried (with stems on)
- 1/2 cup dark chocolate chips or dark chocolate (70% cocoa or higher)
- 1 teaspoon coconut oil (optional, for smoother chocolate)

Instructions:

1. **Prepare the Strawberries:**
   - o Wash the strawberries thoroughly and pat them dry with a paper towel. Make sure the strawberries are completely dry, as any water can cause the chocolate to seize up.
2. **Melt the Chocolate:**
   - o In a microwave-safe bowl, combine the dark chocolate chips or chopped dark chocolate with the coconut oil (if using). Microwave in 20-30 second intervals, stirring after each interval, until the chocolate is fully melted and smooth. Alternatively, you can melt the chocolate in a heatproof bowl set over a pot of simmering water (double boiler method).
3. **Dip the Strawberries:**
   - o Hold each strawberry by the stem and dip it into the melted chocolate, swirling to coat it evenly. Allow any excess chocolate to drip back into the bowl.
4. **Set the Chocolate:**
   - o Place the chocolate-covered strawberries on a parchment-lined baking sheet. If desired, you can add toppings like a sprinkle of sea salt, chopped nuts, or a drizzle of white chocolate while the dark chocolate is still wet.
5. **Chill the Strawberries:**
   - o Place the baking sheet in the refrigerator for about 15-20 minutes, or until the chocolate is fully set and firm.

Day 5

Breakfast: Overnight Oats with Chia Seeds and Almond Milk

Ingredients:

- 1/2 cup rolled oats
- 1 tablespoon chia seeds
- 1/2 cup unsweetened almond milk (or your preferred dairy-free milk)
- 1/4 cup Greek yogurt (optional, for added creaminess)
- 1 tablespoon honey or maple syrup (optional, for added sweetness)
- 1/2 teaspoon vanilla extract (optional)
- Fresh fruit for topping (such as berries, banana slices, or diced apple)
- A sprinkle of nuts or seeds (such as almonds, walnuts, or sunflower seeds)

Instructions:

1. **Combine Ingredients:**
   - In a mason jar or a small bowl, combine the rolled oats, chia seeds, and almond milk. If using Greek yogurt, honey or maple syrup, and vanilla extract, add them to the mixture as well. Stir well to ensure all ingredients are evenly combined.
2. **Refrigerate Overnight:**
   - Cover the jar or bowl with a lid or plastic wrap and refrigerate overnight (or for at least 4-6 hours). This allows the oats to soak up the liquid and the chia seeds to expand, creating a creamy, pudding-like consistency.
3. **Prepare Toppings:**
   - Before serving, prepare your desired toppings. Fresh fruit, nuts, and seeds add flavor, texture, and additional nutrients to your overnight oats.
4. **Serve and Garnish:**
   - In the morning, remove the oats from the refrigerator. Give them a good stir to ensure everything is well mixed. Add your choice of toppings, such as fresh fruit and a sprinkle of nuts or seeds.

Lunch: Roasted Vegetable and Quinoa Bowl

Ingredients:

- 1 cup quinoa, rinsed
- 2 cups water or low-sodium vegetable broth
- 1 zucchini, diced
- 1 red bell pepper, diced
- 1 yellow bell pepper, diced
- 1 red onion, diced
- 1 cup cherry tomatoes, halved
- 1 cup broccoli florets
- 2 tablespoons olive oil
- 1 teaspoon dried oregano
- 1 teaspoon dried basil
- Salt and pepper to taste
- 1/4 cup feta cheese, crumbled (optional)
- 2 tablespoons fresh parsley, chopped (optional)
- Lemon wedges (optional, for serving)

Instructions:

1. **Preheat the Oven:**
   - Preheat your oven to 400°F (200°C).
2. **Cook the Quinoa:**
   - In a medium saucepan, bring 2 cups of water or vegetable broth to a boil. Add the rinsed quinoa, reduce the heat to low, cover, and simmer for about 15 minutes or until the quinoa is tender and the liquid is absorbed. Remove from heat and let sit, covered, for 5 minutes, then fluff with a fork.
3. **Prepare the Vegetables:**
   - While the quinoa is cooking, prepare the vegetables. Dice the zucchini, red and yellow bell peppers, and red onion. Halve the cherry tomatoes and cut the broccoli into florets.
4. **Roast the Vegetables:**
   - Place the diced vegetables and broccoli florets on a large baking sheet. Drizzle with olive oil and sprinkle with dried oregano, dried basil, salt, and pepper. Toss to coat the vegetables evenly.
   - Roast the vegetables in the preheated oven for 20-25 minutes, or until they are tender and lightly browned, stirring halfway through the cooking time.
5. **Assemble the Bowl:**
   - In a large bowl, combine the cooked quinoa and roasted vegetables. Toss gently to mix the ingredients.
6. **Add Toppings (Optional):**
   - Top the quinoa and vegetable mixture with crumbled feta cheese, if using, and garnish with fresh parsley.

Dinner: Lemon Herb Chicken with Cauliflower Rice

Ingredients:

For the Lemon Herb Chicken:

- 2 boneless, skinless chicken breasts
- 2 tablespoons olive oil
- 2 cloves garlic, minced
- Juice of 1 lemon
- 1 tablespoon lemon zest
- 1 teaspoon dried oregano
- 1 teaspoon dried thyme
- Salt and pepper to taste
- Fresh parsley or basil, chopped (optional, for garnish)
- Lemon wedges (optional, for serving)

For the Cauliflower Rice:

- 1 medium head of cauliflower, cut into florets
- 1 tablespoon olive oil
- Salt and pepper to taste
- 1/4 teaspoon garlic powder (optional)
- 1/4 teaspoon onion powder (optional)
- 1 tablespoon fresh parsley, chopped (optional, for garnish)

Instructions:

1. **Prepare the Marinade for the Chicken:**
   - In a small bowl, whisk together the olive oil, minced garlic, lemon juice,

lemon zest, dried oregano, dried thyme, salt, and pepper.

2. **Marinate the Chicken:**
   o Place the chicken breasts in a resealable plastic bag or shallow dish. Pour the marinade over the chicken, making sure it's well coated. Seal the bag or cover the dish, and let the chicken marinate in the refrigerator for at least 30 minutes, or up to 2 hours for maximum flavor.
3. **Prepare the Cauliflower Rice:**
   o While the chicken is marinating, prepare the cauliflower rice. Pulse the cauliflower florets in a food processor until they resemble rice grains. Alternatively, you can grate the cauliflower using a box grater.
4. **Cook the Chicken:**
   o Preheat a large skillet or grill pan over medium-high heat. Remove the chicken from the marinade and discard the excess marinade.
   o Cook the chicken breasts for about 5-7 minutes per side, or until fully cooked through and the internal temperature reaches 165°F (75°C). The chicken should be golden brown and slightly charred on the outside. Remove the chicken from the pan and let it rest for a few minutes before slicing.
5. **Cook the Cauliflower Rice:**
   o In a separate large skillet, heat the olive oil over medium heat. Add the cauliflower rice and sauté for about 5-7 minutes, or until tender. Season with salt, pepper, garlic powder, and onion powder, if using. Stir occasionally to ensure even cooking.
6. **Serve the Meal:**
   o Slice the lemon herb chicken and serve it over a bed of cauliflower rice. Garnish with fresh parsley or basil and add a lemon wedge on the side for extra flavor, if desired.

Snack: Mixed Nuts and Seeds

Ingredients:

- 1/4 cup almonds
- 1/4 cup walnuts
- 1/4 cup cashews
- 2 tablespoons pumpkin seeds (pepitas)
- 2 tablespoons sunflower seeds
- 2 tablespoons dried cranberries or raisins (optional, for added sweetness)
- A pinch of sea salt (optional)

Instructions:

1. **Prepare the Ingredients:**
   o Measure out all the nuts and seeds. If desired, you can lightly toast the nuts and seeds in a dry skillet over medium heat for 3-5 minutes, stirring frequently until they are golden and fragrant. Let them cool completely before mixing.
2. **Mix the Nuts and Seeds:**
   o In a small bowl or airtight container, combine the almonds, walnuts, cashews, pumpkin seeds, and sunflower seeds. Add dried cranberries or raisins for a touch of natural sweetness, if using.
3. **Season (Optional):**
   o If you prefer a slightly salty snack, add a pinch of sea salt and toss the mixture to coat evenly.
4. **Store and Serve:**
   o Store the mixed nuts and seeds in an airtight container at room temperature for up to two weeks. Serve a small portion as a satisfying snack.

Dessert: Apple Slices with Cinnamon Yogurt Dip

Ingredients:

- 2 medium apples (such as Honeycrisp, Fuji, or Gala), cored and sliced
- 1 cup plain Greek yogurt (or dairy-free alternative)

Instructions:

1. **Prepare the Apples:**
   - Wash the apples thoroughly and core them. Slice the apples into thin wedges or rounds. Set aside on a serving plate.
2. **Make the Cinnamon Yogurt Dip:**
   - In a small bowl, combine the Greek yogurt, honey or maple syrup, ground cinnamon, and vanilla extract (if using). Mix well until all ingredients are fully incorporated and the dip is smooth.

- 1 tablespoon honey or maple syrup
- 1/2 teaspoon ground cinnamon
- 1/4 teaspoon vanilla extract (optional)
- A pinch of nutmeg (optional, for extra warmth)

3. **Add Extra Flavor (Optional):**
   - For an extra hint of warmth and flavor, add a pinch of nutmeg to the yogurt dip and stir to combine.
4. **Serve the Dessert:**
   - Place the cinnamon yogurt dip in a small bowl and arrange it on the serving plate alongside the apple slices.

Day 6

Breakfast: Banana Pancakes with Maple Syrup

Ingredients:

- 1 ripe banana, mashed
- 2 large eggs
- 1/4 teaspoon vanilla extract (optional)
- 1/4 teaspoon ground cinnamon (optional)
- 1/4 teaspoon baking powder (optional, for fluffier pancakes)

- Pinch of salt
- 1 tablespoon coconut oil or butter, for cooking
- Maple syrup, for serving
- Fresh fruit, such as berries or banana slices (optional, for topping)

Instructions:

1. **Prepare the Batter:**
   - In a medium bowl, mash the ripe banana until smooth. Add the eggs, vanilla extract, ground cinnamon, baking powder (if using), and a pinch of salt. Whisk until well combined and a smooth batter form.
2. **Heat the Skillet:**
   - Heat a non-stick skillet or griddle over medium heat. Add a small amount of coconut oil or butter to the skillet to coat the surface.
3. **Cook the Pancakes:**
   - Pour a small amount of batter (about 2 tablespoons) onto the skillet for each pancake. Cook for about 2-3 minutes, or until bubbles form on the surface and the edges start to set. Carefully flip the pancakes with a spatula and cook for an additional 1-2 minutes, or until golden brown and cooked through.
4. **Keep Pancakes Warm:**
   - Transfer the cooked pancakes to a plate and cover them with a clean towel to keep them warm while you cook the remaining batter.
5. **Serve the Pancakes:**
   - Stack the pancakes on a plate and drizzle with maple syrup. Top with

fresh fruit, such as berries or banana slices, if desired.

Lunch: Tuna Salad with Mixed Greens

Ingredients:

- 1 can (5 ounces) tuna, drained (preferably packed in water)
- 1 tablespoon Greek yogurt or mayonnaise (for a creamier texture)
- 1 tablespoon Dijon mustard
- 1 celery stalk, finely chopped
- 1/4 red onion, finely chopped
- 1 tablespoon fresh parsley, chopped
- 1 tablespoon lemon juice
- Salt and pepper to taste
- 4 cups mixed salad greens (such as spinach, arugula, and lettuce)
- 1/2 cup cherry tomatoes, halved
- 1/4 cucumber, sliced
- 1/4 avocado, sliced
- 1 tablespoon olive oil (optional, for dressing)
- Additional lemon wedges (optional, for serving)

Instructions:

1. **Prepare the Tuna Salad:**
   - In a medium bowl, combine the drained tuna, Greek yogurt or mayonnaise, Dijon mustard, celery, red onion, parsley, and lemon juice. Mix well until all ingredients are fully combined. Season with salt and pepper to taste.
2. **Prepare the Salad Greens:**
   - In a large mixing bowl, combine the mixed salad greens, cherry tomatoes, and cucumber. Toss gently to mix.
3. **Assemble the Salad:**
   - Place a generous portion of the mixed greens on each serving plate. Top with a scoop of the tuna salad. Add slices of avocado on the side.
4. **Dress the Salad (Optional):**
   - Drizzle the salad with a small amount of olive oil if desired. You can also add a squeeze of fresh lemon juice for extra flavor.

Dinner: Baked Cod with Sweet Potato Fries

Ingredients:

For the Baked Cod:

- 2 cod fillets (about 4-6 ounces each)
- 1 tablespoon olive oil
- 1 teaspoon lemon zest
- Juice of 1/2 lemon
- 1 clove garlic, minced

For the Sweet Potato Fries:

- 2 medium sweet potatoes, peeled and cut into fries
- 1 tablespoon olive oil
- 1/2 teaspoon paprika

- 1 teaspoon dried thyme or parsley
- Salt and pepper to taste
- Lemon wedges (optional, for serving)
- Fresh parsley, chopped (optional, for garnish)

- 1/2 teaspoon garlic powder
- Salt and pepper to taste

Instructions:

1. **Preheat the Oven:**
   - Preheat your oven to 425°F (220°C). Line a baking sheet with parchment paper.
2. **Prepare the Sweet Potato Fries:**
   - In a large bowl, toss the sweet potato fries with olive oil, paprika, garlic powder, salt, and pepper until evenly coated.
   - Spread the sweet potato fries in a single layer on the prepared baking sheet. Bake in the preheated oven for 20-25 minutes, flipping halfway through, until they are crispy and golden brown.
3. **Prepare the Cod Fillets:**
   - While the sweet potato fries are baking, prepare the cod. Place the cod fillets on a separate baking sheet lined with parchment paper.
   - Drizzle the fillets with olive oil and lemon juice. Sprinkle with lemon zest, minced garlic, dried thyme or parsley, salt, and pepper.
4. **Bake the Cod:**
   - Place the baking sheet with the cod fillets in the oven during the last 10-12 minutes of the sweet potato fries' cooking time. Bake the cod for 10-12 minutes, or until the fish is opaque and flakes easily with a fork.
5. **Serve the Meal:**
   - Divide the baked cod and sweet potato fries among plates. Garnish the cod with fresh parsley and serve with lemon wedges on the side, if desired.

Snack: Sliced Bell Peppers with Guacamole

Ingredients:

- 1 red bell pepper, sliced into strips

- 1 yellow bell pepper, sliced into strips
- 1 green bell pepper, sliced into strips

For the Guacamole:

- 1 ripe avocado, peeled and pitted
- 1/4 red onion, finely chopped

- 1/2 small tomato, diced
- 1 tablespoon fresh cilantro, chopped
- Juice of 1/2 lime

- Salt and pepper to taste
- A pinch of cayenne pepper or paprika (optional, for a bit of heat)

Instructions:

1. **Prepare the Bell Peppers:**
   - Wash the bell peppers thoroughly. Cut them in half, remove the seeds and membranes, and slice them into strips. Set aside on a serving plate.
2. **Make the Guacamole:**
   - In a medium bowl, mash the avocado with a fork until smooth (or leave it slightly chunky if you prefer). Add the chopped red onion, diced tomato, cilantro, and lime juice. Mix well until all ingredients are combined.
   - Season the guacamole with salt and pepper to taste. If you like a bit of heat, add a pinch of cayenne pepper or paprika and stir to combine.
3. **Serve the Snack:**
   - Place the guacamole in a small serving bowl and set it on the plate with the sliced bell peppers.

Dessert: Mango Sorbet

Ingredients:

- 3 cups ripe mango chunks (fresh or frozen)
- 1/4 cup water
- 2 tablespoons honey or maple syrup (optional, for added sweetness)
- 1 tablespoon lime juice (optional, for a tangy flavor)
- Fresh mint leaves (optional, for garnish)

Instructions:

1. **Prepare the Mango:**
   - If using fresh mango, peel and pit the mangoes and cut the flesh into chunks. If using frozen mango chunks, allow them to thaw slightly for easier blending.
2. **Blend the Ingredients:**
   - In a blender or food processor, combine the mango chunks, water, honey or maple syrup (if using), and lime juice (if using). Blend until smooth and creamy. If the mixture is too thick, add a bit more water, one tablespoon at a time, to reach the desired consistency.
3. **Freeze the Sorbet:**
   - Pour the mango mixture into a shallow, freezer-safe container. Smooth the top with a spatula. Cover the container and place it in the freezer for at least 2-3 hours, or until the sorbet is firm.
4. **Serve the Sorbet:**
   - Once the mango sorbet is fully frozen, remove it from the freezer and let it sit at room temperature for a few minutes to soften slightly. Scoop the sorbet into bowls or cups.

Day 7

Breakfast: Avocado Toast with Poached Egg

Ingredients:

- 2 slices whole grain or sourdough bread
- 1 ripe avocado
- 1 teaspoon lemon juice
- Salt and pepper to taste
- 2 large eggs

Instructions:

- 1 tablespoon white vinegar (optional, for poaching eggs)
- Red pepper flakes (optional, for garnish)
- Fresh herbs, such as chives or parsley, chopped (optional, for garnish)

1. **Prepare the Avocado Spread:**
   - Cut the ripe avocado in half, remove the pit, and scoop the flesh into a small bowl. Mash the avocado with a fork until smooth. Add the lemon juice, and season with salt and pepper to taste. Set aside.
2. **Toast the Bread:**
   - Toast the slices of whole grain or sourdough bread in a toaster or under a broiler until golden and crispy.
3. **Poach the Eggs:**
   - Fill a medium saucepan with water and bring it to a gentle simmer over medium heat. Add the white vinegar to the water (this helps the egg whites coagulate quickly).
   - Crack one egg into a small bowl or cup. Create a gentle whirlpool in the simmering water with a spoon, then carefully slide the egg into the center of the whirlpool. Poach the egg for about 3-4 minutes for a runny yolk, or longer if you prefer a firmer yolk. Remove the poached egg with a slotted spoon and set it on a plate lined with paper towels to drain. Repeat with the second egg.
4. **Assemble the Avocado Toast:**
   - Spread the mashed avocado evenly over each slice of toasted bread.
5. **Add the Poached Eggs:**
   - Place a poached egg on top of each slice of avocado toast.
6. **Garnish and Serve:**
   - Sprinkle with red pepper flakes, fresh herbs, and additional salt and pepper, if desired.

Lunch: Grilled Vegetable Panini

Ingredients:

- 1 small zucchini, sliced into thin rounds
- 1 small eggplant, sliced into thin rounds
- 1/2 red bell pepper, sliced into strips
- 1/2 yellow bell pepper, sliced into strips
- 1/4 red onion, thinly sliced
- 1 tablespoon olive oil

- Salt and pepper to taste
- 4 slices whole grain or sourdough bread
- 2 tablespoons hummus (or pesto, for added flavor)
- 1/2 cup fresh spinach leaves
- 1/4 cup mozzarella cheese, shredded (optional, for a cheesy panini)

Instructions:

1. **Preheat the Grill or Panini Press:**
   - Preheat a grill, grill pan, or panini press over medium-high heat.
2. **Prepare the Vegetables:**
   - In a bowl, toss the zucchini, eggplant, red and yellow bell peppers, and red onion with olive oil, salt, and pepper until evenly coated.

3. **Grill the Vegetables:**
   - Place the vegetables on the preheated grill or grill pan. Cook for 3-4 minutes on each side, or until they are tender and have nice grill marks. Remove the vegetables from the grill and set them aside.

4. **Assemble the Panini:**
   - Spread a layer of hummus (or pesto) on one side of each slice of bread. On two of the slices, layer the grilled vegetables, fresh spinach leaves, and shredded mozzarella cheese (if using).

5. **Top and Grill the Panini:**
   - Place the remaining two slices of bread on top of the layered vegetables, hummus side down, to form a sandwich. Place the sandwiches on the preheated grill or panini press and cook for 3-5 minutes, or until the bread is golden and crispy and the cheese (if using) is melted.

6. **Serve the Panini:**
   - Remove the panini from the grill or press and let them cool slightly. Slice each panini in half.

Dinner: Stuffed Bell Peppers with Lean Ground Turkey

Ingredients:

- 4 large bell peppers (any color), tops cut off and seeds removed
- 1-pound lean ground turkey
- 1 tablespoon olive oil
- 1 small onion, diced
- 2 cloves garlic, minced
- 1 medium zucchini, diced
- 1 cup cooked quinoa or brown rice
- 1 can (15 ounces) diced tomatoes, drained
- 1 teaspoon dried oregano
- 1 teaspoon dried basil
- 1/2 teaspoon paprika
- Salt and pepper to taste
- 1/2 cup shredded mozzarella or cheddar cheese (optional, for topping)
- Fresh parsley or cilantro, chopped (optional, for garnish)

Instructions:

1. **Preheat the Oven:**
   - Preheat your oven to 375°F (190°C). Place the bell peppers upright in a baking dish and set aside.

2. **Cook the Filling:**
   - In a large skillet, heat the olive oil over medium heat. Add the diced onion and cook for about 3-4 minutes until it becomes translucent. Add the minced garlic and cook for an additional 1 minute until fragrant.

3. **Add the Ground Turkey:**
   - Add the lean ground turkey to the skillet and cook, breaking it up with a spoon, until it is browned and fully cooked, about 5-7 minutes.

4. **Add Vegetables and Seasonings:**
   - Stir in the diced zucchini, cooked quinoa or brown rice, diced tomatoes, dried oregano, dried basil, paprika, salt, and pepper. Cook for an additional 5 minutes, or until the zucchini is tender and the flavors are well combined. Remove the skillet from heat.

5. **Stuff the Bell Peppers:**
   - Spoon the turkey and vegetable mixture evenly into the hollowed-out bell peppers, filling them to the top.

6. **Bake the Stuffed Peppers:**
   - Cover the baking dish with aluminum foil and bake in the preheated oven for 30 minutes. Remove the foil and sprinkle the tops of the stuffed peppers with shredded cheese, if using. Bake for an additional 10-15 minutes, or until the cheese is melted and bubbly and the peppers are tender.

7. **Serve and Garnish:**
   - Remove the stuffed bell peppers from the oven and let them cool slightly. Garnish with chopped fresh parsley or cilantro, if desired.

Snack: Fruit Smoothie with Protein Powder

Ingredients:

- 1/2 cup frozen mixed berries (such as strawberries, blueberries, and raspberries)
- 1/2 banana, sliced
- 1/2 cup unsweetened almond milk (or your preferred dairy-free milk)
- 1/4 cup Greek yogurt (or a dairy-free alternative)
- 1 scoop protein powder (vanilla or unflavored)
- 1 teaspoon honey or maple syrup (optional, for added sweetness)
- A handful of ice cubes (optional, for a thicker smoothie)

Instructions:

1. **Prepare the Ingredients:**
   - Slice the banana and measure out the frozen mixed berries, almond milk, Greek yogurt, and protein powder.
2. **Blend the Smoothie:**
   - In a blender, combine the frozen berries, banana, almond milk, Greek yogurt, protein powder, and honey or maple syrup (if using). Add a handful of ice cubes for a thicker, colder smoothie if desired.
3. **Blend Until Smooth:**
   - Blend on high until all the ingredients are fully combined and the smoothie is smooth and creamy. If the smoothie is too thick, add a bit more almond milk until you reach your desired consistency.
4. **Serve and Enjoy:**
   - Pour the smoothie into a glass and serve immediately.

Dessert: Coconut Macaroons

Ingredients:

- 2 1/2 cups unsweetened shredded coconut
- 2/3 cup sweetened condensed milk
- 1 teaspoon vanilla extract
- 2 large egg whites
- 1/4 teaspoon salt
- Optional: 1/2 cup dark chocolate chips (for drizzling or dipping)

Instructions:

1. **Preheat the Oven:**
   - Preheat your oven to 325°F (160°C).

Line a baking sheet with parchment paper.

2. **Mix the Coconut Mixture:**
   o In a large mixing bowl, combine the shredded coconut, sweetened condensed milk, and vanilla extract. Stir until the coconut is fully coated and the mixture is sticky.

3. **Prepare the Egg Whites:**
   o In a separate clean bowl, whisk the egg whites and salt until stiff peaks form. This should take about 2-3 minutes with a hand mixer or a few minutes longer if whisking by hand.

4. **Fold the Egg Whites:**
   o Gently fold the beaten egg whites into the coconut mixture. Be careful not to deflate the egg whites, which helps give the macaroons a light and airy texture.

5. **Form the Macaroons:**
   o Using a spoon or a small ice cream scoop, drop heaping tablespoons of the mixture onto the prepared baking sheet, spacing them about 1 inch apart.

6. **Bake the Macaroons:**
   o Bake in the preheated oven for 20-25 minutes, or until the tops are golden brown and the macaroons are set. Keep an eye on them to prevent burning.

7. **Cool the Macaroons:**
   o Remove the macaroons from the oven and let them cool on the baking sheet for a few minutes before transferring them to a wire rack to cool completely.

8. **Optional Chocolate Drizzle or Dip:**
   o If you want to add a chocolate touch, melt the dark chocolate chips in a microwave-safe bowl in 30-second intervals, stirring in between, until smooth. Drizzle the melted chocolate over the cooled macaroons or dip the bottoms in the chocolate and let them set on a parchment-lined tray until the chocolate hardens.

Week 2: Building Up Flavor and Variety

Day 8

Breakfast: Chia Pudding with Mango and Coconut

Ingredients:

- 1/4 cup chia seeds
- 1 cup unsweetened coconut milk (from a carton, not canned)
- 1 tablespoon honey or maple syrup (optional, for added sweetness)
- 1/2 teaspoon vanilla extract (optional)
- 1/2 ripe mango, diced
- 2 tablespoons unsweetened shredded coconut
- Fresh mint leaves (optional, for garnish)

Instructions:

1. **Prepare the Chia Pudding:**
   o In a medium bowl or mason jar, combine the chia seeds, coconut milk, honey or maple syrup (if using), and vanilla extract (if using). Stir well to ensure the chia seeds are evenly distributed and not clumping together.

2. **Refrigerate the Pudding:**
   o Cover the bowl or jar and refrigerate for at least 2 hours or overnight. The chia seeds will absorb the coconut milk and expand, creating a thick, pudding-like consistency.

3. **Prepare the Toppings:**
   o While the chia pudding is setting, dice the mango and set it aside. Measure out the shredded coconut as well.

4. **Assemble the Chia Pudding:**

- Once the chia pudding has set, give it a good stir to ensure an even texture. Divide the pudding into serving bowls or glasses.
5. **Add Toppings and Garnish:**
   - Top each bowl of chia pudding with diced mango and a sprinkle of shredded coconut. For an extra touch, garnish with fresh mint leaves.

Lunch: Spinach and Feta Stuffed Chicken Breast

Ingredients:

- 2 boneless, skinless chicken breasts
- Salt and pepper to taste
- 1 tablespoon olive oil
- 1 cup fresh spinach leaves, chopped
- 1/4 cup feta cheese, crumbled
- 1/4 teaspoon garlic powder
- 1/4 teaspoon dried oregano
- 1/4 teaspoon dried basil
- 1/4 cup sun-dried tomatoes, chopped (optional)
- Toothpicks, for securing the chicken

Instructions:

1. **Preheat the Oven:**
   - Preheat your oven to 375°F (190°C). Lightly grease a baking dish with olive oil or cooking spray.
2. **Prepare the Chicken Breasts:**
   - Carefully slice each chicken breast horizontally to create a pocket, being careful not to cut all the way through. Season both sides of the chicken breasts with salt and pepper.
3. **Prepare the Stuffing:**
   - In a small bowl, combine the chopped spinach, crumbled feta cheese, garlic powder, dried oregano, dried basil, and sun-dried tomatoes (if using). Mix well until all the ingredients are evenly distributed.
4. **Stuff the Chicken Breasts:**
   - Spoon the spinach and feta mixture into the pocket of each chicken breast. Use toothpicks to secure the opening and keep the stuffing inside.
5. **Sear the Chicken:**
   - In a large ovenproof skillet, heat the olive oil over medium heat. Add the stuffed chicken breasts and sear for 3-4 minutes on each side, or until golden brown.
6. **Bake the Chicken:**
   - Transfer the skillet to the preheated oven and bake for 20-25 minutes, or until the chicken is cooked through and the internal temperature reaches 165°F (75°C).
7. **Remove and Rest:**
   - Remove the skillet from the oven and let the chicken rest for a few minutes. Remove the toothpicks carefully before serving.

Dinner: Vegetarian Chili with Kidney Beans

Ingredients:

- 1 tablespoon olive oil
- 1 medium onion, diced
- 2 cloves garlic, minced
- 1 red bell pepper, diced
- 1 green bell pepper, diced
- 1 medium zucchini, diced
- 1 medium carrot, diced
- 1 can (15 ounces) kidney beans, drained and rinsed
- 1 can (15 ounces) black beans, drained and rinsed
- 1 can (15 ounces) diced tomatoes
- 1 can (15 ounces) tomato sauce
- 1 cup vegetable broth
- 2 tablespoons tomato paste
- 1 tablespoon chili powder
- 1 teaspoon ground cumin
- 1 teaspoon paprika
- 1/2 teaspoon ground coriander
- 1/2 teaspoon dried oregano
- Salt and pepper to taste
- 1/4 teaspoon cayenne pepper (optional, for heat)
- Fresh cilantro, chopped (optional, for garnish)
- Sliced avocado (optional, for topping)

Instructions:

1. **Sauté the Vegetables:**
   - In a large pot or Dutch oven, heat the olive oil over medium heat. Add the diced onion and cook for 3-4 minutes until softened. Add the minced garlic and cook for an additional 1 minute until fragrant.
2. **Add the Vegetables:**
   - Add the diced red bell pepper, green bell pepper, zucchini, and carrot to the pot. Cook for 5-7 minutes, stirring occasionally, until the vegetables begin to soften.
3. **Add the Beans and Tomatoes:**
   - Add the kidney beans, black beans, diced tomatoes, tomato sauce, vegetable broth, and tomato paste to the pot. Stir well to combine.
4. **Season the Chili:**
   - Add the chili powder, ground cumin, paprika, ground coriander, dried oregano, salt, pepper, and cayenne pepper (if using) to the pot. Stir to incorporate all the spices evenly.
5. **Simmer the Chili:**
   - Bring the chili to a simmer over medium-high heat. Once simmering, reduce the heat to low and cover the pot. Let the chili simmer for 20-30 minutes, stirring occasionally, until the flavors meld and the vegetables are tender.
6. **Adjust Seasoning:**
   - Taste the chili and adjust the seasoning as needed with additional salt, pepper, or spices.
7. **Serve and Garnish:**
   - Ladle the vegetarian chili into bowls. Garnish with chopped fresh cilantro and sliced avocado, if desired.

Snack: Edamame with Sea Salt

Ingredients:

- 1 cup edamame (fresh or frozen, in the pod)
- 1/2 teaspoon sea salt (or to taste)

Instructions:

1. **Cook the Edamame:**
   - Bring a pot of water to a boil over medium-high heat. Add the edamame to the boiling water and cook for 3-5

minutes, or until the edamame pods are bright green and tender. If using frozen edamame, follow the package instructions for cooking time.

2. **Drain the Edamame:**
   o   Drain the cooked edamame in a colander and shake off any excess water. You can also rinse them briefly under cold water to stop the cooking process and cool them slightly.

3. **Season with Sea Salt:**
   o   Transfer the cooked edamame to a serving bowl. Sprinkle with sea salt, tossing the pods gently to ensure even seasoning.

Dessert: Blueberry Yogurt Parfait

Ingredients:

- 1 cup plain Greek yogurt (or dairy-free yogurt alternative)
- 1/2 cup fresh or frozen blueberries
- 2 tablespoons honey or maple syrup (optional, for added sweetness)
- 1/4 cup granola (choose a low-sugar variety)
- 1 tablespoon chia seeds or flaxseeds (optional, for added fiber)
- Fresh mint leaves (optional, for garnish)

Instructions:

1. **Prepare the Blueberries:**
   o   If using frozen blueberries, let them thaw slightly. If using fresh blueberries, rinse them under cold water and pat them dry with a paper towel.

2. **Layer the Parfait:**
   o   In a glass or bowl, add a few spoonsful of Greek yogurt to create the first layer. Drizzle with a small amount of honey or maple syrup, if desired.
   o   Add a layer of blueberries on top of the yogurt, followed by a sprinkle of granola and chia seeds or flaxseeds, if using.

3. **Repeat the Layers:**
   o   Continue layering the yogurt, honey or maple syrup, blueberries, granola, and seeds until all ingredients are used, finishing with a layer of blueberries and granola on top.

4. **Garnish and Serve:**
   o   Garnish with fresh mint leaves, if desired, for an extra touch of flavor and color.

Day 9

Breakfast: Buckwheat Pancakes with Fresh Strawberries

Ingredients:

- 1/2 cup buckwheat flour
- 1/2 cup whole wheat flour (or a gluten-free alternative)
- 1 tablespoon baking powder
- 1 tablespoon sugar or honey (optional, for added sweetness)
- 1/4 teaspoon salt

- 1 cup milk (dairy or dairy-free alternative)
- 1 large egg
- 1 tablespoon melted butter or coconut oil
- 1 teaspoon vanilla extract (optional)
- 1 cup fresh strawberries, sliced
- Maple syrup (optional, for serving)
- Additional butter or coconut oil (for cooking)

Instructions:

1. **Prepare the Batter:**
   - In a medium mixing bowl, whisk together the buckwheat flour, whole wheat flour, baking powder, sugar (if using), and salt.
2. **Mix Wet Ingredients:**
   - In a separate bowl, whisk together the milk, egg, melted butter or coconut oil, and vanilla extract (if using) until well combined.
3. **Combine Wet and Dry Ingredients:**
   - Pour the wet ingredients into the dry ingredients and stir gently until just combined. Be careful not to overmix; a few lumps are okay.
4. **Heat the Skillet:**
   - Heat a non-stick skillet or griddle over medium heat. Add a small amount of butter or coconut oil to the skillet to coat the surface.
5. **Cook the Pancakes:**
   - Pour about 1/4 cup of batter onto the skillet for each pancake. Cook for 2-3 minutes, or until bubbles form on the surface and the edges begin to set. Flip the pancakes and cook for an additional 1-2 minutes, or until golden brown and cooked through.
6. **Keep Pancakes Warm:**
   - Transfer the cooked pancakes to a plate and cover them with a clean towel to keep them warm while you cook the remaining batter.
7. **Serve the Pancakes:**
   - Stack the buckwheat pancakes on a plate and top with fresh strawberry slices. Drizzle with maple syrup if desired.

Lunch: Salmon and Avocado Salad

Ingredients:

- 4-6 ounces of cooked salmon (grilled, baked, or canned)
- 4 cups mixed salad greens (such as spinach, arugula, and lettuce)
- 1 ripe avocado, sliced
- 1/2 cucumber, sliced
- 1/2 cup cherry tomatoes, halved
- 1/4 red onion, thinly sliced

- 1/4 cup feta cheese, crumbled (optional)
- 2 tablespoons olive oil
- 1 tablespoon lemon juice
- 1 teaspoon Dijon mustard
- Salt and pepper to taste
- Fresh dill or parsley, chopped (optional, for garnish)

Instructions:

1. **Prepare the Salmon:**
   - If using fresh salmon, cook it by grilling or baking until fully cooked and flaky. Let it cool slightly before

flaking it into bite-sized pieces. If using canned salmon, drain and flake it with a fork.

2. **Prepare the Salad Base:**
   o In a large mixing bowl, combine the mixed salad greens, sliced cucumber, cherry tomatoes, and red onion.

3. **Add the Salmon and Avocado:**
   o Add the flaked salmon and sliced avocado to the salad. Gently toss to combine, being careful not to mash the avocado.

4. **Make the Dressing:**
   o In a small bowl, whisk together the olive oil, lemon juice, Dijon mustard, salt, and pepper until well combined. Adjust seasoning to taste.

5. **Dress the Salad:**
   o Drizzle the dressing over the salad and toss gently to coat all the ingredients evenly.

6. **Add Optional Toppings:**
   o Sprinkle the salad with crumbled feta cheese if using, and garnish with fresh dill or parsley for added flavor and color.

Dinner: Baked Chicken with Quinoa and Broccoli

Ingredients:

For the Baked Chicken:

- 2 boneless, skinless chicken breasts
- 1 tablespoon olive oil
- 2 cloves garlic, minced
- 1 teaspoon dried thyme
- 1 teaspoon dried rosemary
- 1 teaspoon paprika
- Salt and pepper to taste
- Juice of 1/2 lemon

For the Quinoa and Broccoli:

- 1 cup quinoa, rinsed
- 2 cups water or low-sodium chicken broth
- 2 cups broccoli florets
- 1 tablespoon olive oil
- Salt and pepper to taste
- 1/2 teaspoon garlic powder (optional)
- 1/4 teaspoon red pepper flakes (optional, for a bit of heat)

Instructions:

1. **Preheat the Oven:**
   o Preheat your oven to 375°F (190°C). Lightly grease a baking dish with olive oil or cooking spray.

2. **Prepare the Chicken:**

o   In a small bowl, mix together the olive oil, minced garlic, dried thyme, dried rosemary, paprika, salt, pepper, and lemon juice.
o   Rub the seasoning mixture all over the chicken breasts, ensuring they are well coated.

3. **Bake the Chicken:**
o   Place the seasoned chicken breasts in the prepared baking dish. Bake in the preheated oven for 25-30 minutes, or until the chicken is cooked through and the internal temperature reaches 165°F (75°C).

4. **Cook the Quinoa:**
o   While the chicken is baking, prepare the quinoa. In a medium saucepan, bring 2 cups of water or chicken broth to a boil. Add the rinsed quinoa, reduce the heat to low, cover, and simmer for about 15 minutes, or until the quinoa is tender and the liquid is absorbed.

o   Remove from heat and let it sit, covered, for 5 minutes. Fluff with a fork.

5. **Steam or Roast the Broccoli:**
o   For steaming: Bring a pot of water to a boil and place a steamer basket over it. Add the broccoli florets to the steamer basket, cover, and steam for 5-7 minutes until tender.
o   For roasting: Toss the broccoli florets in olive oil, salt, pepper, garlic powder (if using), and red pepper flakes (if using). Spread on a baking sheet and roast in the oven at 375°F (190°C) for 15-20 minutes, or until tender and slightly crispy.

6. **Combine and Serve:**
o   Slice the baked chicken breasts and serve them over a bed of quinoa with a side of broccoli. Drizzle with extra lemon juice or garnish with fresh herbs, if desired.

Snack: Apple Slices with Almond Butter

Ingredients:

- 1 medium apple (such as Fuji, Honeycrisp, or Gala)
- 2 tablespoons almond butter (unsweetened and smooth)
- A sprinkle of cinnamon (optional)
- A drizzle of honey (optional, for added sweetness)
- A handful of chopped nuts (such as walnuts or almonds, optional, for extra crunch)

Instructions:

1. **Prepare the Apple:**
o   Wash the apple thoroughly under running water. Core the apple and cut it into thin slices.

2. **Serve with Almond Butter:**
o   Arrange the apple slices on a plate. Serve with a small bowl or spoonful of almond butter on the side for dipping.

3. **Add Extra Flavor (Optional):**
o   For added flavor, sprinkle the apple slices with a bit of cinnamon. Drizzle with honey for extra sweetness, and top with chopped nuts for added crunch, if desired.

Dessert: Peach Cobbler

Ingredients:

For the Filling:

- 4 cups fresh peaches, peeled and sliced (or use frozen peaches, thawed)
- 1/4 cup honey or maple syrup (adjust to taste)
- 1 tablespoon lemon juice
- 1/2 teaspoon ground cinnamon
- 1/4 teaspoon ground nutmeg (optional)
- 1 tablespoon cornstarch or arrowroot powder (for thickening)

For the Topping:

- 1 cup whole wheat flour (or gluten-free flour blend)
- 1/4 cup rolled oats
- 2 tablespoons sugar or coconut sugar
- 1 teaspoon baking powder
- 1/4 teaspoon salt
- 1/4 cup cold unsalted butter or coconut oil, cut into small pieces
- 1/2 cup milk (dairy or dairy-free alternative)

Instructions:

1. **Preheat the Oven:**
   - Preheat your oven to 375°F (190°C). Lightly grease a baking dish or pie pan with a bit of butter or coconut oil.
2. **Prepare the Peach Filling:**
   - In a large bowl, combine the sliced peaches, honey or maple syrup, lemon juice, cinnamon, nutmeg (if using), and cornstarch. Toss gently to coat the peaches evenly. Pour the peach mixture into the prepared baking dish.
3. **Prepare the Cobbler Topping:**
   - In a separate bowl, combine the whole wheat flour, rolled oats, sugar, baking powder, and salt. Add the cold butter or coconut oil pieces and use a pastry cutter or your fingers to work the butter into the dry ingredients until the mixture resembles coarse crumbs.
4. **Add Milk to the Topping:**
   - Gradually stir in the milk until the topping mixture is just moistened and a soft dough form. Be careful not to overmix.
5. **Assemble the Cobbler:**
   - Spoon the topping mixture evenly over the peaches in the baking dish. The topping should cover most of the fruit but doesn't need to be perfectly even.
6. **Bake the Cobbler:**
   - Bake in the preheated oven for 30-35 minutes, or until the topping is golden brown and the peach filling is bubbling around the edges.
7. **Cool Slightly and Serve:**
   - Remove the peach cobbler from the oven and let it cool slightly before serving. This will help the filling set.

Day 10

Breakfast: Smoothie with Kale, Pineapple, and Ginger

Ingredients:

- 1 cup fresh kale leaves, stems removed and chopped
- 1/2 cup fresh or frozen pineapple chunks
- 1/2 ripe banana
- 1/2 teaspoon fresh ginger, grated
- 1 cup unsweetened almond milk (or your preferred dairy-free milk)
- 1 tablespoon chia seeds or flaxseeds (optional, for added fiber)

- 1 tablespoon honey or maple syrup (optional, for added sweetness)

Instructions:

1. **Prepare the Ingredients:**
   o Wash and chop the kale leaves. Measure out the pineapple chunks, banana, and grated ginger.
2. **Blend the Smoothie:**
   o In a blender, combine the chopped kale, pineapple chunks, banana, grated

- A handful of ice cubes (optional, for a colder smoothie)

ginger, almond milk, and chia seeds or flaxseeds (if using). Add honey or maple syrup for sweetness, if desired.

3. **Add Ice and Blend Until Smooth:**
   o Add a handful of ice cubes for a thicker, colder smoothie if desired. Blend on high until all the ingredients are fully combined and the smoothie is smooth and creamy.

Lunch: Turkey and Cheese Lettuce Wraps

Ingredients:

- 8 large lettuce leaves (such as romaine, iceberg, or butter lettuce)
- 8 slices deli turkey breast (low sodium, preferably)
- 4 slices cheese (such as Swiss, cheddar, or provolone)
- 1/2 avocado, sliced

- 1/2 cup cucumber, sliced into thin sticks
- 1/2 cup cherry tomatoes, halved
- 1/4 red onion, thinly sliced (optional)
- 2 tablespoons hummus or Greek yogurt (optional, for added flavor)
- Salt and pepper to taste

Instructions:

1. **Prepare the Lettuce Leaves:**
   o Wash and dry the lettuce leaves thoroughly. Lay them flat on a clean surface or plate.
2. **Assemble the Wraps:**
   o Spread a small amount of hummus or Greek yogurt on each lettuce leaf for added flavor (if using).
   o Layer each lettuce leaf with a slice of deli turkey, a slice of cheese, a few slices of avocado, cucumber sticks,

cherry tomatoes, and red onion (if using). Season with salt and pepper to taste.

3. **Roll the Wraps:**
   o Carefully roll each lettuce leaf around the filling, folding in the sides as you go to create a wrap. Use a toothpick to secure the wrap if needed.

4. **Serve and Enjoy:**
   o Arrange the lettuce wraps on a plate and serve immediately.

Dinner: Sautéed Shrimp with Zoodles and Pesto

Ingredients:

- 1-pound large shrimp, peeled and deveined

- 2 tablespoons olive oil, divided
- 2 cloves garlic, minced

- 1/4 teaspoon red pepper flakes (optional, for a bit of heat)
- Salt and pepper to taste
- 3 medium zucchinis, spiralized into noodles (zoodles)
- 1/2 cup pesto sauce (store-bought or homemade)
- 1/4 cup cherry tomatoes, halved (optional)
- Fresh basil leaves, chopped (optional, for garnish)
- Lemon wedges (optional, for serving)

Instructions:

1. **Prepare the Zoodles:**
   - Spiralize the zucchinis into noodles using a spiralizer. Set the zoodles aside.
2. **Cook the Shrimp:**
   - Heat 1 tablespoon of olive oil in a large skillet over medium heat. Add the minced garlic and red pepper flakes (if using) and sauté for about 30 seconds until fragrant.
   - Add the shrimp to the skillet in a single layer. Season with salt and pepper. Cook the shrimp for about 2-3 minutes per side, or until they are pink and opaque. Remove the shrimp from the skillet and set aside.
3. **Sauté the Zoodles:**
   - In the same skillet, add the remaining tablespoon of olive oil. Add the zoodles and sauté for about 2-3 minutes, or until they are tender but still slightly crisp. Be careful not to overcook the zoodles, as they can become mushy.
4. **Combine with Pesto:**
   - Reduce the heat to low. Add the pesto sauce to the skillet with the zoodles and toss to coat the zoodles evenly in the sauce.
5. **Add the Shrimp and Tomatoes:**
   - Return the cooked shrimp to the skillet and add the cherry tomatoes (if using). Toss everything together gently to combine and heat through for about 1-2 minutes.
6. **Serve and Garnish:**
   - Divide the sautéed shrimp and zoodles among serving plates. Garnish with fresh basil leaves and serve with lemon wedges on the side, if desired.

Snack: Rice Cakes with Peanut Butter and Banana

Ingredients:

- 2 rice cakes (plain or lightly salted)
- 2 tablespoons peanut butter (unsweetened and natural)
- 1 medium banana, sliced
- A sprinkle of cinnamon (optional, for extra flavor)
- A drizzle of honey (optional, for added sweetness)
- A handful of chia seeds or flaxseeds (optional, for added crunch and nutrition)

Instructions:

1. **Prepare the Rice Cakes:**
   - Place the rice cakes on a clean plate or flat surface.
2. **Spread the Peanut Butter:**
   - Spread 1 tablespoon of peanut butter evenly over each rice cake.
3. **Add Banana Slices:**
   - Top each rice cake with banana slices, arranging them evenly over the peanut butter.
4. **Add Optional Toppings:**

o Sprinkle a little cinnamon over the banana slices for extra flavor. Drizzle with honey for added sweetness, if desired. You can also sprinkle some chia seeds or flaxseeds for a nutritional boost.

Dessert: Chocolate Avocado Mousse

Ingredients:

- 2 ripe avocados, peeled and pitted
- 1/4 cup unsweetened cocoa powder
- 1/4 cup honey, maple syrup, or agave syrup (adjust to taste)
- 1/4 cup almond milk (or your preferred dairy-free milk)
- 1 teaspoon vanilla extract
- A pinch of salt
- Fresh berries (such as raspberries or strawberries) for garnish (optional)
- Dark chocolate shavings or cacao nibs for garnish (optional)
- Whipped coconut cream (optional, for serving)

Instructions:

1. **Prepare the Avocados:**
   o Cut the ripe avocados in half, remove the pits, and scoop the flesh into a blender or food processor.
2. **Blend the Mousse Ingredients:**
   o Add the unsweetened cocoa powder, honey or maple syrup, almond milk, vanilla extract, and a pinch of salt to the blender or food processor with the avocado.
3. **Blend Until Smooth:**
   o Blend all the ingredients together until the mixture is completely smooth and creamy. You may need to stop and scrape down the sides a few times to ensure everything is well combined. If the mousse is too thick, add a little more almond milk, one tablespoon at a time, until you reach your desired consistency.
4. **Taste and Adjust:**
   o Taste the mousse and adjust the sweetness if needed by adding more honey or maple syrup.
5. **Chill the Mousse:**
   o Transfer the mousse to individual serving dishes or bowls. Refrigerate for at least 30 minutes to 1 hour to allow the flavors to meld and the mousse to firm up slightly.
6. **Serve and Garnish:**
   o Before serving, garnish the chocolate avocado mousse with fresh berries, dark chocolate shavings, or cacao nibs, if desired. You can also add a dollop of whipped coconut cream for extra indulgence.

Day 11

Breakfast: Greek Yogurt with Honey and Granola

Ingredients:

- 1 cup plain Greek yogurt (or a dairy-free yogurt alternative)
- 2 tablespoons honey
- 1/4 cup granola (choose a low-sugar variety)
- 1/2 cup fresh berries (such as blueberries, strawberries, or raspberries)

- 1 tablespoon nuts (such as almonds or walnuts, optional)
- 1 tablespoon chia seeds or flaxseeds (optional, for added fiber)

Instructions:

1. **Prepare the Yogurt:**
   o Scoop the Greek yogurt into a serving bowl.
2. **Add Honey and Toppings:**
   o Drizzle the honey over the yogurt. Top with granola, fresh berries, nuts, and

- A sprinkle of cinnamon (optional, for extra flavor)

seeds (if using). Sprinkle a little cinnamon on top for extra flavor, if desired.

3. **Mix and Serve:**
   o Gently mix the yogurt with the toppings to combine or leave them layered for added texture.

Lunch: Vegetable Soup with Whole Grain Crackers

Ingredients:

For the Vegetable Soup:

- 1 tablespoon olive oil
- 1 medium onion, diced
- 2 cloves garlic, minced
- 2 carrots, diced
- 2 celery stalks, diced
- 1 medium zucchini, diced
- 1 cup green beans, trimmed and cut into 1-inch pieces
- 1 can (15 ounces) diced tomatoes
- 4 cups low-sodium vegetable broth

- 1 teaspoon dried thyme
- 1 teaspoon dried basil
- 1/2 teaspoon dried oregano
- Salt and pepper to taste
- 1 cup baby spinach leaves
- 1/4 cup fresh parsley, chopped (optional, for garnish)
- 1/2 lemon, juiced (optional, for added brightness)

For Serving:

- Whole grain crackers (choose a low-sodium variety)

Instructions:

1. **Sauté the Aromatics:**
   o In a large pot or Dutch oven, heat the olive oil over medium heat. Add the

diced onion and sauté for 3-4 minutes, until softened. Add the minced garlic and cook for an additional 1 minute until fragrant.

2. **Add the Vegetables:**

o   Add the carrots, celery, zucchini, and green beans to the pot. Sauté for 5-6 minutes, stirring occasionally, until the vegetables begin to soften.

3. **Add the Tomatoes and Broth:**
   o   Pour in the diced tomatoes (with their juices) and the vegetable broth. Stir to combine. Add the dried thyme, dried basil, dried oregano, salt, and pepper. Bring the soup to a simmer over medium-high heat.

4. **Simmer the Soup:**
   o   Once the soup reaches a simmer, reduce the heat to low and cover the pot. Let the soup simmer for 20-25 minutes, or until the vegetables are tender and the flavors have melded together.

5. **Add Spinach and Adjust Seasoning:**
   o   Stir in the baby spinach leaves and cook for an additional 2-3 minutes until wilted. Taste the soup and adjust the seasoning with more salt, pepper, or lemon juice if desired.

6. **Serve the Soup:**
   o   Ladle the vegetable soup into bowls and garnish with fresh parsley, if using.

7. **Serve with Crackers:**
   o   Serve the soup hot with a side of whole grain crackers for added crunch and fiber.

Dinner: Beef and Broccoli Stir-Fry

Ingredients:

- 1-pound lean beef (such as flank steak or sirloin), thinly sliced against the grain
- 3 cups broccoli florets
- 2 tablespoons olive oil, divided
- 2 cloves garlic, minced
- 1 tablespoon fresh ginger, minced
- 1/4 cup low-sodium soy sauce or tamari (for gluten-free option)
- 1 tablespoon oyster sauce (optional, for added flavor)
- 1 tablespoon honey or maple syrup
- 1 tablespoon cornstarch or arrowroot powder (for thickening)
- 1/4 cup water or low-sodium beef broth
- 1 teaspoon sesame oil (optional, for added flavor)
- 1/4 teaspoon red pepper flakes (optional, for a bit of heat)
- 1 tablespoon sesame seeds (optional, for garnish)
- 2 green onions, sliced (optional, for garnish)
- Cooked brown rice or quinoa, for serving

Instructions:

1. **Prepare the Beef:**
   o   Thinly slice the beef against the grain. In a small bowl, mix 1 tablespoon of olive oil, minced garlic, minced ginger, soy sauce, oyster sauce (if using), honey or maple syrup, and cornstarch or arrowroot powder. Add the beef slices to the bowl and toss to coat. Let marinate for 15-20 minutes while you prepare the rest of the ingredients.

2. **Prepare the Broccoli:**
   o   Steam or blanch the broccoli florets in boiling water for 2-3 minutes until tender but still crisp. Drain and set aside.

3. **Cook the Beef:**
   o   In a large skillet or wok, heat the remaining 1 tablespoon of olive oil over medium-high heat. Add the marinated beef slices in a single layer and cook for about 2-3 minutes, or until the beef is browned and cooked through. Remove the beef from the skillet and set aside.

4. **Make the Stir-Fry Sauce:**
   o   In a small bowl, mix the water or beef broth with the sesame oil (if using) and red pepper flakes (if using). Pour this

mixture into the skillet, scraping up any browned bits from the bottom of the pan.

5. **Add Broccoli and Beef to the Skillet:**
   - Add the steamed broccoli florets and cooked beef back to the skillet. Stir to combine and cook for an additional 2-3 minutes, or until everything is heated through and the sauce has thickened.
6. **Serve the Stir-Fry:**
   - Divide the beef and broccoli stir-fry among plates. Garnish with sesame seeds and sliced green onions if desired.
7. **Serve with Rice or Quinoa:**
   - Serve the stir-fry hot over a bed of cooked brown rice or quinoa.

Snack: Cucumber Slices with Tzatziki

Ingredients:

- 1 large cucumber, sliced into rounds
- 1 cup plain Greek yogurt (or dairy-free yogurt alternative)
- 1/2 cup grated cucumber (about half a small cucumber, peeled and seeded)
- 1 clove garlic, minced
- 1 tablespoon fresh dill, chopped
- 1 tablespoon fresh lemon juice
- 1 tablespoon olive oil
- Salt and pepper to taste
- A pinch of paprika (optional, for garnish)
- Fresh dill or mint leaves (optional, for garnish)

Instructions:

1. **Prepare the Tzatziki Sauce:**
   - In a medium bowl, combine the grated cucumber, Greek yogurt, minced garlic, chopped dill, lemon juice, olive oil, salt, and pepper. Mix well until all ingredients are fully incorporated. Adjust seasoning to taste.
2. **Chill the Tzatziki:**
   - Cover the bowl and refrigerate the tzatziki sauce for at least 15 minutes to allow the flavors to meld together.
3. **Prepare the Cucumber Slices:**
   - Wash the cucumber thoroughly and slice it into thin rounds. Arrange the cucumber slices on a serving plate.
4. **Serve with Tzatziki:**
   - Place the chilled tzatziki sauce in a small bowl and set it on the plate with the cucumber slices.
5. **Garnish and Serve:**
   - Garnish the tzatziki with a sprinkle of paprika and a few fresh dill or mint leaves, if desired.

Dessert: Baked Apple with Oats and Cinnamon

Ingredients:

- 2 medium apples (such as Honeycrisp, Granny Smith, or Fuji)
- 1/4 cup rolled oats
- 2 tablespoons chopped nuts (such as walnuts or almonds)
- 2 tablespoons raisins or dried cranberries (optional)
- 1 teaspoon ground cinnamon
- 1 tablespoon honey or maple syrup
- 1 tablespoon melted butter or coconut oil
- 1/2 teaspoon vanilla extract (optional)
- A pinch of salt
- Greek yogurt or whipped cream (optional, for serving)

Instructions:

1. **Preheat the Oven:**
   - Preheat your oven to 350°F (175°C). Lightly grease a small baking dish with butter or coconut oil.
2. **Prepare the Apples:**
   - Wash the apples thoroughly. Cut off the top of each apple (about 1/4 inch) and set aside. Use a paring knife or an apple corer to remove the core and seeds, creating a hollow center in each apple. Be careful not to cut through the bottom of the apple.
3. **Prepare the Filling:**
   - In a small bowl, combine the rolled oats, chopped nuts, raisins or dried cranberries (if using), ground cinnamon, honey or maple syrup, melted butter or coconut oil, vanilla extract (if using), and a pinch of salt. Mix well until all ingredients are evenly coated.
4. **Stuff the Apples:**
   - Spoon the oat mixture into the hollowed-out centers of the apples, pressing down gently to pack the filling. Place the stuffed apples in the prepared baking dish. If desired, drizzle a little extra honey or maple syrup over the top of the apples.
5. **Bake the Apples:**
   - Place the baking dish in the preheated oven and bake for 25-30 minutes, or until the apples are tender and the filling is golden and bubbling. The apples should be soft but not mushy.
6. **Serve the Baked Apples:**
   - Remove the baked apples from the oven and let them cool slightly. Serve warm with a dollop of Greek yogurt or whipped cream, if desired.

Day 12

Breakfast: Almond Butter Smoothie with Dates and Cocoa

Ingredients:

- 1 cup unsweetened almond milk (or your preferred dairy-free milk)
- 2 tablespoons almond butter
- 2-3 Medjool dates, pitted
- 1 tablespoon unsweetened cocoa powder
- 1/2 frozen banana
- 1/2 teaspoon vanilla extract (optional)
- A pinch of cinnamon (optional)
- A handful of ice cubes (optional, for a colder smoothie)

Instructions:

1. **Prepare the Ingredients:**
   - Pit the Medjool dates and slice them into smaller pieces for easier blending.

Measure out the almond butter, cocoa powder, and other ingredients.

2. **Blend the Smoothie:**
   - In a blender, combine the almond milk, almond butter, pitted dates, unsweetened cocoa powder, frozen banana, vanilla extract (if using), and cinnamon (if using).
3. **Add Ice and Blend Until Smooth:**
   - If you prefer a colder, thicker smoothie, add a handful of ice cubes. Blend on high until all the ingredients are fully combined and the smoothie is smooth and creamy.
4. **Serve and Enjoy:**
   - Pour the smoothie into a glass and serve immediately.

Lunch: Grilled Chicken Caesar Salad

Ingredients:

For the Salad:

- 2 boneless, skinless chicken breasts
- 1 tablespoon olive oil
- Salt and pepper to taste
- 1 head of romaine lettuce, chopped
- 1/4 cup grated Parmesan cheese
- 1/2 cup cherry tomatoes, halved (optional)
- 1/4 cup whole grain croutons (optional)

For the Caesar Dressing:

- 1/2 cup Greek yogurt (or dairy-free yogurt alternative)
- 1 tablespoon lemon juice
- 1 teaspoon Dijon mustard
- 1 teaspoon Worcestershire sauce
- 1 clove garlic, minced
- 2 tablespoons grated Parmesan cheese
- Salt and pepper to taste
- 1-2 tablespoons water (to thin the dressing, if needed)

Instructions:

1. **Prepare the Chicken:**
   - Preheat a grill or grill pan over medium-high heat. Drizzle the chicken breasts with olive oil and season with salt and pepper.
2. **Grill the Chicken:**
   - Place the chicken breasts on the grill and cook for about 6-7 minutes per side, or until the chicken is cooked through and has reached an internal temperature of 165°F (75°C). Remove the chicken from the grill and let it rest for a few minutes before slicing it into thin strips.
3. **Prepare the Dressing:**
   - In a small bowl, whisk together the Greek yogurt, lemon juice, Dijon mustard, Worcestershire sauce, minced garlic, grated Parmesan cheese, salt, and pepper. Add a little water to thin the dressing to your desired consistency, if needed.
4. **Assemble the Salad:**
   - In a large salad bowl, add the chopped romaine lettuce. Top with the sliced grilled chicken, grated Parmesan cheese, cherry tomatoes (if using), and whole grain croutons (if using).
5. **Dress the Salad:**
   - Drizzle the Caesar dressing over the salad and toss gently to coat all the ingredients evenly.

6. **Serve and Enjoy:**

- o   Divide the salad into portions and serve immediately.

Dinner: Vegetable and Tofu Stir-Fry

Ingredients:

- 1 block (14 ounces) firm or extra-firm tofu, drained and cubed
- 2 tablespoons soy sauce or tamari (for gluten-free option)
- 1 tablespoon sesame oil (or olive oil), divided
- 1 tablespoon cornstarch or arrowroot powder
- 1 red bell pepper, sliced
- 1 yellow bell pepper, sliced
- 1 medium zucchini, sliced into half-moons
- 1 cup broccoli florets
- 1 cup snap peas or green beans
- 2 cloves garlic, minced
- 1 tablespoon fresh ginger, minced
- 1/4 cup low-sodium vegetable broth or water
- 2 tablespoons hoisin sauce or teriyaki sauce (optional, for added flavor)
- 1 teaspoon rice vinegar or apple cider vinegar (optional, for tanginess)
- 1/4 teaspoon red pepper flakes (optional, for heat)
- 1 tablespoon sesame seeds (optional, for garnish)
- Cooked brown rice or quinoa, for serving
- Fresh cilantro or green onions, chopped (optional, for garnish)

Instructions:

1. **Prepare the Tofu:**
   - o   Drain the tofu and pat it dry with a paper towel to remove excess moisture. Cut the tofu into cubes. In a bowl, toss the tofu cubes with 1 tablespoon of soy sauce or tamari and cornstarch until evenly coated.
2. **Cook the Tofu:**
   - o   Heat 1/2 tablespoon of sesame oil in a large skillet or wok over medium-high heat. Add the tofu cubes in a single layer and cook for 4-5 minutes on each side, or until golden and crispy. Remove the tofu from the skillet and set aside.
3. **Sauté the Vegetables:**
   - o   In the same skillet, add the remaining 1/2 tablespoon of sesame oil. Add the minced garlic and ginger, and sauté for about 30 seconds until fragrant.
   - o   Add the sliced bell peppers, zucchini, broccoli florets, and snap peas or green beans. Stir-fry the vegetables for 5-7 minutes, or until they are tender-crisp.
4. **Prepare the Stir-Fry Sauce:**
   - o   In a small bowl, mix together the vegetable broth, remaining 1 tablespoon of soy sauce or tamari, hoisin sauce or teriyaki sauce (if using), rice vinegar (if using), and red pepper flakes (if using).
5. **Combine Tofu and Vegetables:**
   - o   Add the cooked tofu back into the skillet with the vegetables. Pour the stir-fry sauce over the tofu and vegetables. Toss everything together to coat evenly and cook for an additional 2-3 minutes, or until the sauce is heated through and slightly thickened.
6. **Serve the Stir-Fry:**
   - o   Divide the vegetable and tofu stir-fry among serving plates. Garnish with sesame seeds, fresh cilantro, or green onions if desired.
7. **Serve with Rice or Quinoa:**
   - o   Serve the stir-fry hot over a bed of cooked brown rice or quinoa for a complete meal.

Snack: Mixed Berries with Whipped Coconut Cream

Ingredients:

- 1 cup mixed berries (such as strawberries, blueberries, raspberries, and blackberries)
- 1 can (14 ounces) full-fat coconut milk or coconut cream, chilled overnight
- 1-2 tablespoons powdered sugar or honey (optional, for sweetness)
- 1/2 teaspoon vanilla extract (optional, for flavor)
- Fresh mint leaves (optional, for garnish)

Instructions:

1. **Prepare the Berries:**
   - Wash and pat dry the mixed berries. Arrange them in a serving bowl or individual cups.
2. **Prepare the Coconut Cream:**
   - Open the chilled can of coconut milk or coconut cream. Scoop out the solidified cream that has separated from the liquid into a mixing bowl. Discard the liquid or save it for another use.
3. **Whip the Coconut Cream:**
   - Using a hand mixer or a whisk, whip the coconut cream on medium speed until it becomes fluffy and light, about 2-3 minutes. Add powdered sugar or honey and vanilla extract (if using) and continue to whip until fully incorporated and smooth.
4. **Serve the Berries with Coconut Cream:**
   - Spoon the whipped coconut cream over the mixed berries.
5. **Garnish and Serve:**
   - Garnish with fresh mint leaves if desired and serve immediately.

Dessert: Lemon Sorbet

Ingredients:

- 1 cup freshly squeezed lemon juice (about 4-5 lemons)
- 1 cup water
- 3/4 cup granulated sugar or honey (adjust to taste)
- 1 tablespoon lemon zest
- Fresh mint leaves (optional, for garnish)

Instructions:

1. **Make the Simple Syrup:**
   - In a small saucepan, combine the water and granulated sugar or honey. Heat over medium heat, stirring constantly, until the sugar is fully dissolved. Remove from heat and let the syrup cool to room temperature.
2. **Prepare the Lemon Mixture:**
   - In a large bowl, combine the freshly squeezed lemon juice and lemon zest. Once the simple syrup has cooled, add it to the lemon mixture and stir well to combine.
3. **Chill the Mixture:**

    o   Cover the bowl with plastic wrap and refrigerate the lemon mixture for at least 1 hour, or until thoroughly chilled.

4. **Churn the Sorbet:**
   - o Pour the chilled lemon mixture into an ice cream maker and churn according to the manufacturer's instructions until the sorbet reaches a smooth, soft-serve consistency. This usually takes about 20-30 minutes.

5. **Freeze the Sorbet:**
   - o Transfer the churned sorbet to an airtight container and freeze for at least 2 hours, or until firm.

6. **Serve the Sorbet:**
   - o Scoop the lemon sorbet into bowls or cups. Garnish with fresh mint leaves if desired.

Day 13

Breakfast: Sweet Potato and Egg Hash

Ingredients:

- 1 medium sweet potato, peeled and diced into small cubes
- 1 tablespoon olive oil
- 1/2 red bell pepper, diced
- 1/2 green bell pepper, diced
- 1/2 small onion, diced
- 2 cloves garlic, minced
- Salt and pepper to taste
- 1/2 teaspoon smoked paprika (optional, for added flavor)
- 1/4 teaspoon ground cumin (optional, for added flavor)
- 2 large eggs
- Fresh parsley or cilantro, chopped (optional, for garnish)
- Hot sauce (optional, for serving)

Instructions:

1. **Cook the Sweet Potatoes:**
   - o Heat the olive oil in a large skillet over medium heat. Add the diced sweet potatoes and cook for about 10 minutes, stirring occasionally, until they start to soften and turn golden brown.

2. **Add the Vegetables:**
   - o Add the diced red and green bell peppers and onion to the skillet. Cook for another 5-7 minutes, or until the vegetables are tender and the sweet potatoes are fully cooked. Add the minced garlic and cook for an additional 1-2 minutes, stirring frequently, until fragrant.

3. **Season the Hash:**
   - o Season the sweet potato and vegetable mixture with salt, pepper, smoked paprika, and ground cumin (if using). Stir well to combine and cook for another minute to let the flavors meld together.

4. **Create Space for the Eggs:**
   - o Use a spoon to make two small wells in the sweet potato mixture. Crack an egg into each well.

5. **Cook the Eggs:**
   - o Reduce the heat to low, cover the skillet with a lid, and cook the eggs until the whites are set but the yolks are still runny, about 3-5 minutes. For firmer yolks, cook for an additional 1-2 minutes.

6. **Garnish and Serve:**
   - o Remove the skillet from the heat and garnish with fresh parsley or cilantro if desired. Add a few dashes of hot sauce for a bit of heat, if using.

Lunch: Quinoa and Black Bean Salad

Ingredients:

- 1 cup quinoa, rinsed
- 2 cups water or low-sodium vegetable broth
- 1 can (15 ounces) black beans, drained and rinsed
- 1 cup cherry tomatoes, halved
- 1/2 red bell pepper, diced
- 1/2 yellow bell pepper, diced
- 1/2 red onion, finely chopped
- 1 cup corn kernels (fresh, frozen, or canned)
- 1/4 cup fresh cilantro, chopped
- 1 avocado, diced (optional)

For the Dressing:

- 1/4 cup olive oil
- 2 tablespoons lime juice (about 1-2 limes)
- 1 tablespoon red wine vinegar
- 1 teaspoon ground cumin
- Salt and pepper to taste

Instructions:

1. **Cook the Quinoa:**
   - In a medium saucepan, bring 2 cups of water or vegetable broth to a boil. Add the rinsed quinoa, reduce the heat to low, cover, and simmer for about 15 minutes, or until the quinoa is tender and the liquid is absorbed. Remove from heat and let it sit, covered, for 5 minutes. Fluff with a fork and set aside to cool.
2. **Prepare the Vegetables:**
   - While the quinoa is cooking, prepare the vegetables. Halve the cherry tomatoes, dice the red and yellow bell peppers, finely chop the red onion, and drain and rinse the black beans. If using fresh corn, cut the kernels off the cob; if using frozen, thaw it; if using canned, drain it.
3. **Make the Dressing:**
   - In a small bowl, whisk together the olive oil, lime juice, red wine vinegar, ground cumin, salt, and pepper until well combined.
4. **Combine the Salad Ingredients:**
   - In a large mixing bowl, combine the cooked quinoa, black beans, cherry tomatoes, red and yellow bell peppers, red onion, corn, and fresh cilantro.
5. **Add the Dressing:**
   - Pour the dressing over the quinoa and vegetable mixture. Toss gently to ensure everything is evenly coated with the dressing.
6. **Add Avocado (Optional):**
   - If using, gently fold in the diced avocado.
7. **Serve and Enjoy:**
   - Serve the quinoa and black bean salad chilled or at room temperature.

Dinner: Baked Halibut with Green Beans

Ingredients:

For the Baked Halibut:

- 2 halibut filets (about 6 ounces each)
- 2 tablespoons olive oil
- 2 cloves garlic, minced

- 1 tablespoon lemon juice
- 1 teaspoon lemon zest
- 1 teaspoon dried thyme
- Salt and pepper to taste
- Lemon wedges (optional, for serving)

For the Green Beans:

- 1-pound fresh green beans, trimmed
- 1 tablespoon olive oil
- 1/2 teaspoon garlic powder

Instructions:

1. **Preheat the Oven:**
   - Preheat your oven to 400°F (200°C). Line a baking sheet with parchment paper or lightly grease it with olive oil.
2. **Prepare the Halibut:**
   - In a small bowl, mix the olive oil, minced garlic, lemon juice, lemon zest, dried thyme, salt, and pepper. Place the halibut fillets on the prepared baking sheet. Brush the olive oil mixture over the fillets, coating them evenly.
3. **Bake the Halibut:**
   - Bake the halibut in the preheated oven for 12-15 minutes, or until the fish is opaque and flakes easily with a fork. The baking time may vary depending on the thickness of the fillets.

- Fresh parsley or dill, chopped (optional, for garnish)

- Salt and pepper to taste
- 1/4 teaspoon red pepper flakes (optional, for a bit of heat

4. **Prepare the Green Beans:**
   - While the halibut is baking, prepare the green beans. In a mixing bowl, toss the green beans with olive oil, garlic powder, salt, pepper, and red pepper flakes (if using).
5. **Roast the Green Beans:**
   - Spread the green beans in a single layer on a separate baking sheet. Place them in the oven during the last 10 minutes of the halibut's baking time. Roast for 10 minutes, or until the green beans are tender and slightly caramelized.
6. **Serve the Halibut and Green Beans:**
   - Remove the halibut and green beans from the oven. Transfer the baked halibut to serving plates and add the roasted green beans on the side.
7. **Garnish and Serve:**
   - Garnish the halibut with fresh parsley or dill, if desired, and serve with lemon wedges on the side for an extra burst of flavor.

Snack: Roasted Chickpeas

Ingredients:

- 1 can (15 ounces) chickpeas, drained and rinsed
- 1 tablespoon olive oil
- 1/2 teaspoon salt
- 1/2 teaspoon garlic powder

Instructions:

1. **Preheat the Oven:**

- 1/2 teaspoon paprika
- 1/4 teaspoon ground cumin (optional)
- 1/4 teaspoon black pepper
- A pinch of cayenne pepper (optional, for a bit of heat)

   - Preheat your oven to 400°F (200°C). Line a baking sheet with parchment paper.

2. **Prepare the Chickpeas:**
   o After draining and rinsing the chickpeas, spread them out on a clean kitchen towel or paper towels. Pat them dry thoroughly to remove any excess moisture, which helps them roast evenly and become crispy.
3. **Season the Chickpeas:**
   o In a large bowl, toss the dried chickpeas with olive oil, salt, garlic powder, paprika, ground cumin (if using), black pepper, and cayenne pepper (if using). Ensure the chickpeas are evenly coated with the oil and spices.
4. **Roast the Chickpeas:**
   o Spread the seasoned chickpeas in a single layer on the prepared baking sheet. Roast in the preheated oven for 20-30 minutes, shaking the pan halfway through the cooking time to ensure even roasting. The chickpeas should be golden brown and crispy.
5. **Cool and Serve:**
   o Remove the chickpeas from the oven and let them cool slightly on the baking sheet. They will continue to crisp up as they cool.

Dessert: Pineapple Upside-Down Cake

Ingredients:

For the Topping:

- 1/4 cup unsalted butter, melted
- 1/2 cup brown sugar
- 1 can (20 ounces) pineapple slices in juice, drained
- 10-12 maraschino cherries, drained (optional)

For the Cake Batter:

- 1 1/2 cups all-purpose flour (or a gluten-free flour blend)
- 1/2 cup granulated sugar
- 1/4 cup brown sugar
- 2 teaspoons baking powder
- 1/4 teaspoon salt
- 1/2 cup unsweetened applesauce
- 1/4 cup unsalted butter, melted
- 2 large eggs
- 1 teaspoon vanilla extract
- 1/2 cup milk (dairy or dairy-free alternative)

Instructions:

1. **Preheat the Oven:**
   o Preheat your oven to 350°F (175°C). Grease a 9-inch round cake pan with butter or non-stick cooking spray.
2. **Prepare the Topping:**
   o Pour the melted butter into the bottom of the prepared cake pan. Sprinkle the brown sugar evenly over the butter. Arrange the pineapple slices on top of the brown sugar in a single layer and place a maraschino cherry in the center of each pineapple slice (if using).
3. **Mix the Dry Ingredients:**
   o In a medium bowl, whisk together the flour, granulated sugar, brown sugar, baking powder, and salt.
4. **Mix the Wet Ingredients:**
   o In a separate large bowl, combine the applesauce, melted butter, eggs, vanilla extract, and milk. Whisk until smooth and well combined.

5. **Combine the Wet and Dry Ingredients:**
   o Gradually add the dry ingredients to the wet ingredients, stirring until just combined. Be careful not to overmix; a few lumps are fine.
6. **Pour the Batter:**
   o Pour the batter evenly over the pineapple and brown sugar mixture in the cake pan, spreading it gently to ensure it covers the fruit completely.
7. **Bake the Cake:**
   o Bake in the preheated oven for 35-40 minutes, or until a toothpick inserted into the center of the cake comes out clean and the top is golden brown.
8. **Cool and Invert the Cake:**
   o Allow the cake to cool in the pan for about 10 minutes. Run a knife around the edges to loosen the cake. Place a serving plate upside down over the pan, and carefully invert the pan and plate together. Gently lift the pan off the cake to reveal the pineapple topping.

Day 14

Breakfast: Protein-Packed Omelet with Vegetables

Ingredients:

- 3 large eggs (or 2 eggs and 2 egg whites for lower cholesterol)
- 1/4 cup milk (dairy or dairy-free alternative)
- Salt and pepper to taste
- 1/4 cup diced bell peppers (red, green, or yellow)
- 1/4 cup diced onion
- 1/4 cup cherry tomatoes, halved
- 1/4 cup fresh spinach, chopped
- 1/4 cup mushrooms, sliced
- 1/4 cup shredded low-fat cheese (such as cheddar, mozzarella, or feta)
- 1 tablespoon olive oil or butter
- Fresh herbs, such as parsley or chives, chopped (optional, for garnish)
- Hot sauce or salsa (optional, for serving)

Instructions:

1. **Prepare the Vegetables:**
   o Wash and dice the bell peppers and onion. Halve the cherry tomatoes, chop the spinach, and slice the mushrooms. Set all the vegetables aside.
2. **Whisk the Eggs:**
   o In a small bowl, whisk together the eggs, milk, salt, and pepper until well combined and slightly frothy.
3. **Cook the Vegetables:**
   o Heat the olive oil or butter in a non-stick skillet over medium heat. Add the diced bell peppers, onion, and mushrooms, and sauté for 3-4 minutes until they are softened. Add the cherry tomatoes and spinach, and cook for an additional 1-2 minutes, until the spinach is wilted.
4. **Pour the Egg Mixture:**
   o Pour the egg mixture over the sautéed vegetables in the skillet, ensuring the eggs are evenly distributed. Let the eggs cook undisturbed for about 2-3 minutes, or until the edges start to set.
5. **Add the Cheese:**
   o Sprinkle the shredded cheese evenly over one half of the omelet. Allow the omelet to cook for another 1-2 minutes, or until the eggs are mostly set but still slightly runny on top.
6. **Fold the Omelet:**
   o Using a spatula, gently fold the omelet in half over the cheese. Cook for another 1-2 minutes, or until the cheese is melted and the omelet is cooked through.
7. **Serve and Garnish:**
   o Slide the omelet onto a plate and garnish with fresh herbs if desired. Add a few dashes of hot sauce or a spoonful of salsa for extra flavor, if using.

Lunch: Mediterranean Tuna Salad

Ingredients:

- 2 cans (5 ounces each) tuna in water, drained
- 1/2 cup cherry tomatoes, halved
- 1/2 cucumber, diced
- 1/4 red onion, finely chopped
- 1/4 cup Kalamata olives, pitted and sliced
- 1/4 cup feta cheese, crumbled (optional)
- 2 tablespoons capers, drained
- 2 tablespoons fresh parsley, chopped

- 2 tablespoons fresh basil, chopped (optional)
- 2 tablespoons extra-virgin olive oil
- 1 tablespoon red wine vinegar
- 1 tablespoon lemon juice
- 1 teaspoon Dijon mustard
- Salt and pepper to taste
- Romaine lettuce leaves or mixed greens, for serving

Instructions:

1. **Prepare the Tuna:**
   - Drain the canned tuna and place it in a large mixing bowl. Use a fork to break up the tuna into bite-sized pieces.
2. **Add Vegetables and Mix-Ins:**
   - Add the halved cherry tomatoes, diced cucumber, finely chopped red onion, sliced Kalamata olives, crumbled feta cheese (if using), capers, fresh parsley, and basil (if using) to the bowl with the tuna.
3. **Make the Dressing:**
   - In a small bowl, whisk together the olive oil, red wine vinegar, lemon juice, Dijon mustard, salt, and pepper until well combined.
4. **Combine the Salad:**
   - Pour the dressing over the tuna and vegetable mixture. Gently toss everything together to ensure the ingredients are evenly coated with the dressing.
5. **Serve the Salad:**
   - Serve the Mediterranean tuna salad over a bed of romaine lettuce leaves or mixed greens.

Dinner: Chicken and Spinach Stuffed Mushrooms

Ingredients:

- 8 large portobello or cremini mushrooms, stems removed and cleaned
- 2 tablespoons olive oil, divided
- 1/2-pound ground chicken (or finely chopped cooked chicken breast)
- 2 cloves garlic, minced
- 1/2 small onion, finely chopped
- 2 cups fresh spinach, chopped

- 1/4 cup breadcrumbs (whole wheat or gluten-free)
- 1/4 cup grated Parmesan cheese (optional)
- 1/4 teaspoon red pepper flakes (optional, for a bit of heat)
- Salt and pepper to taste
- 1/4 cup shredded mozzarella cheese (optional, for topping)
- Fresh parsley or basil, chopped (optional, for garnish)

Instructions:

1. **Preheat the Oven:**
   o Preheat your oven to 375°F (190°C). Line a baking sheet with parchment paper or lightly grease it with olive oil.
2. **Prepare the Mushrooms:**
   o Remove the stems from the mushrooms and clean the caps with a damp paper towel to remove any dirt. Arrange the mushroom caps, gill side up, on the prepared baking sheet. Brush the mushroom caps with 1 tablespoon of olive oil and season with a little salt and pepper.
3. **Cook the Chicken Filling:**
   o Heat the remaining 1 tablespoon of olive oil in a skillet over medium heat. Add the minced garlic and chopped onion, and sauté for 2-3 minutes until the onion is soft and translucent. Add the ground chicken and cook for 5-7 minutes, breaking it up with a spoon, until it is fully cooked and no longer pink.
4. **Add Spinach and Seasonings:**
   o Add the chopped spinach to the skillet with the chicken and cook for another 2-3 minutes until the spinach is wilted. Stir in the breadcrumbs, Parmesan cheese (if using), red pepper flakes (if using), salt, and pepper. Mix well to combine all ingredients and remove from heat.
5. **Stuff the Mushrooms:**
   o Spoon the chicken and spinach mixture evenly into each mushroom cap, pressing down gently to fill them completely.
6. **Bake the Stuffed Mushrooms:**
   o Place the stuffed mushrooms in the preheated oven and bake for 15-20 minutes, or until the mushrooms are tender and the filling is heated through.
7. **Add Cheese and Finish Baking:**
   o If using, sprinkle shredded mozzarella cheese over the top of each stuffed mushroom during the last 5 minutes of baking. Continue baking until the cheese is melted and bubbly.
8. **Serve and Garnish:**
   o Remove the mushrooms from the oven and let them cool slightly. Garnish with fresh parsley or basil if desired.

Snack: Trail Mix with Dried Fruit and Nuts

Ingredients:

- 1/2 cup almonds
- 1/2 cup walnuts
- 1/2 cup cashews
- 1/4 cup sunflower seeds or pumpkin seeds (pepitas)
- 1/4 cup raisins or dried cranberries
- 1/4 cup dried apricots, chopped
- 1/4 cup dried apple slices, chopped
- 1/4 cup dark chocolate chips (optional, for added sweetness)
- A pinch of sea salt (optional)

Instructions:

1. **Prepare the Ingredients:**
   o Measure out all the nuts, seeds, dried fruit, and dark chocolate chips (if using). Chop any large pieces of dried fruit into bite-sized pieces for easier mixing and eating.
2. **Mix the Trail Mix:**
   o In a large mixing bowl, combine the almonds, walnuts, cashews, sunflower seeds or pumpkin seeds, raisins or dried cranberries, dried apricots, dried apple slices, and dark chocolate chips (if using).
3. **Season (Optional):**
   o If you prefer a slightly salty snack, add a pinch of sea salt to the mix and toss gently to coat.
4. **Store the Trail Mix:**
   o Transfer the trail mix to an airtight container or resealable plastic bag.

Store at room temperature for up to two
weeks.

Dessert: Raspberry Cheesecake Bites

Ingredients:

For the Crust:

- 1 cup graham cracker crumbs (or gluten-free graham crackers, crushed)
- 2 tablespoons unsalted butter, melted
- 1 tablespoon sugar (optional)

For the Cheesecake Filling:

- 8 ounces cream cheese, softened (regular or reduced fat)
- 1/4 cup Greek yogurt (or dairy-free yogurt alternative)
- 1/4 cup honey or maple syrup
- 1 teaspoon vanilla extract
- 1/2 cup fresh raspberries, mashed

For the Topping:

- Fresh raspberries (for garnish)
- A few mint leaves (optional, for garnish)

Instructions:

1. **Prepare the Crust:**
   - Preheat your oven to 350°F (175°C). Line a mini muffin tin with paper liners or grease it lightly with cooking spray.
   - In a small bowl, combine the graham cracker crumbs, melted butter, and sugar (if using). Mix until the crumbs are evenly coated with butter.
   - Spoon about 1 tablespoon of the crumb mixture into each muffin cup and press down firmly to create a crust. Use the back of a spoon or your fingers to press the crust into an even layer.
2. **Bake the Crust:**
   - Bake the crusts in the preheated oven for about 5 minutes, or until they are set and slightly golden. Remove from the oven and let them cool while you prepare the filling.
3. **Prepare the Cheesecake Filling:**
   - In a medium mixing bowl, beat the softened cream cheese, Greek yogurt, honey or maple syrup, and vanilla extract until smooth and creamy. Fold in the mashed raspberries until well combined.
4. **Fill the Muffin Cups:**
   - Spoon the cheesecake mixture over the cooled crusts in the muffin tin, filling each cup almost to the top.
5. **Chill the Cheesecake Bites:**
   - Refrigerate the cheesecake bites for at least 2-3 hours, or until they are set and firm.
6. **Garnish and Serve:**
   - Once the cheesecake bites are chilled and set, remove them from the muffin tin. Garnish each bite with a fresh raspberry and a mint leaf if desired.

Week 3: Expanding Your Culinary Horizons

Day 15

Breakfast: Smoothie with Almond Milk, Berries, and Spinach

Ingredients:

- 1 cup unsweetened almond milk (or your preferred dairy-free milk)
- 1/2 cup fresh or frozen mixed berries (such as strawberries, blueberries, raspberries)
- 1/2 banana, frozen or fresh
- 1 cup fresh spinach leaves
- 1 tablespoon chia seeds or flaxseeds (optional, for added fiber)
- 1 tablespoon honey or maple syrup (optional, for added sweetness)
- 1/2 teaspoon vanilla extract (optional, for extra flavor)
- A handful of ice cubes (optional, for a thicker, colder smoothie)

Instructions:

1. **Prepare the Ingredients:**
   o Measure out all the ingredients. If using fresh berries, rinse them thoroughly. Peel and slice the banana if using fresh.
2. **Blend the Smoothie:**
   o In a blender, combine the almond milk, mixed berries, banana, spinach leaves, chia seeds or flaxseeds (if using), honey or maple syrup (if using), and vanilla extract (if using).
3. **Add Ice and Blend Until Smooth:**
   o Add a handful of ice cubes for a colder, thicker texture if desired. Blend on high until all ingredients are fully combined and the smoothie is smooth and creamy.
4. **Serve and Enjoy:**
   o Pour the smoothie into a glass and serve immediately.

Lunch: Quinoa and Kale Salad

Ingredients:

- 1 cup quinoa, rinsed
- 2 cups water or low-sodium vegetable broth
- 4 cups kale, stems removed, and leaves chopped
- 1/2 cup cherry tomatoes, halved
- 1/2 cucumber, diced
- 1/4 red onion, thinly sliced
- 1/4 cup feta cheese, crumbled (optional)
- 1/4 cup dried cranberries or raisins
- 1/4 cup toasted almonds or walnuts, chopped

For the Dressing:

- 1/4 cup extra-virgin olive oil
- 2 tablespoons lemon juice
- 1 tablespoon apple cider vinegar
- 1 teaspoon Dijon mustard
- 1 clove garlic, minced
- Salt and pepper to taste

Instructions:

1. **Cook the Quinoa:**
   - In a medium saucepan, bring 2 cups of water or vegetable broth to a boil. Add the rinsed quinoa, reduce the heat to low, cover, and simmer for about 15 minutes, or until the quinoa is tender and the liquid is absorbed. Remove from heat and let it sit, covered, for 5 minutes. Fluff with a fork and set aside to cool.
2. **Prepare the Kale:**
   - While the quinoa is cooking, prepare the kale. Remove the stems and chop the leaves into bite-sized pieces. Place the chopped kale in a large mixing bowl. To soften the kale, drizzle with a small amount of olive oil and a pinch of salt, then gently massage the kale with your hands for 1-2 minutes until it becomes tender and dark green.
3. **Prepare the Vegetables and Mix-Ins:**
   - Add the halved cherry tomatoes, diced cucumber, thinly sliced red onion, crumbled feta cheese (if using), dried cranberries or raisins, and toasted nuts to the bowl with the kale.
4. **Make the Dressing:**
   - In a small bowl, whisk together the olive oil, lemon juice, apple cider vinegar, Dijon mustard, minced garlic, salt, and pepper until well combined.
5. **Combine the Salad Ingredients:**
   - Add the cooked and cooled quinoa to the bowl with the kale and vegetables. Pour the dressing over the salad and toss gently to combine all ingredients evenly.
6. **Serve the Salad:**
   - Divide the quinoa and kale salad among serving plates or bowls.

Dinner: Spaghetti Squash with Marinara Sauce

Ingredients:

For the Spaghetti Squash:

- 1 medium spaghetti squash
- 1 tablespoon olive oil
- Salt and pepper to taste

For the Marinara Sauce:

- 1 tablespoon olive oil
- 1 small onion, finely chopped
- 2 cloves garlic, minced
- 1 can (15 ounces) crushed tomatoes
- 1/2 teaspoon dried basil
- 1/2 teaspoon dried oregano
- 1/4 teaspoon red pepper flakes (optional, for a bit of heat)
- Salt and pepper to taste
- 1 teaspoon sugar or honey (optional, to balance acidity)
- Fresh basil or parsley, chopped (optional, for garnish)

Instructions:

1. **Prepare the Spaghetti Squash:**
   - Preheat your oven to 400°F (200°C).

Line a baking sheet with parchment paper.

- o Cut the spaghetti squash in half lengthwise and scoop out the seeds with a spoon.
- o Drizzle the cut sides of the squash with olive oil and season with salt and pepper.
- o Place the squash halves cut side down on the prepared baking sheet and roast for 35-40 minutes, or until the squash is tender and easily pierced with a fork.

2. **Make the Marinara Sauce:**
   - o While the squash is roasting, heat 1 tablespoon of olive oil in a medium saucepan over medium heat. Add the chopped onion and sauté for 3-4 minutes until softened. Add the minced garlic and sauté for another 1 minute until fragrant.
   - o Add the crushed tomatoes, dried basil, dried oregano, red pepper flakes (if using), salt, pepper, and sugar or honey (if using) to the saucepan. Stir to combine.
   - o Bring the sauce to a simmer and reduce the heat to low. Let the sauce simmer gently for 15-20 minutes, stirring occasionally, to allow the flavors to meld together.

3. **Scrape the Spaghetti Squash:**
   - o Once the squash is done roasting, remove it from the oven and let it cool slightly. Use a fork to scrape the inside of each squash half to create spaghetti-like strands.

4. **Combine the Squash and Sauce:**
   - o Divide the spaghetti squash strands among serving plates. Top each portion with a generous amount of marinara sauce.

5. **Garnish and Serve:**
   - o Garnish with fresh basil or parsley if desired.

Snack: Almond Butter on Whole Grain Crackers

Ingredients:

- 6-8 whole grain crackers (choose a low-sodium, whole wheat, or gluten-free variety)
- 2 tablespoons almond butter (unsweetened and natural)
- 1 teaspoon honey or maple syrup (optional, for added sweetness)
- A sprinkle of chia seeds or flaxseeds (optional, for added nutrition)
- A pinch of cinnamon (optional, for extra flavor)
- Sliced banana or apple (optional, for topping)

Instructions:

1. **Prepare the Crackers:**
   - o Lay out the whole grain crackers on a clean plate or flat surface.
2. **Spread the Almond Butter:**
   - o Spread about 1/2 tablespoon of almond butter evenly over each cracker.
3. **Add Optional Toppings:**
   - o Drizzle a little honey or maple syrup over the almond butter if desired for added sweetness. Sprinkle with chia seeds, flaxseeds, or a pinch of cinnamon for extra nutrition and flavor. If using, top with thin slices of banana or apple for a fresh, fruity addition.

Dessert: Frozen Yogurt with Fresh Fruit

Ingredients:

- 2 cups plain Greek yogurt (or dairy-free yogurt alternative)
- 1/4 cup honey or maple syrup (adjust to taste)
- 1 teaspoon vanilla extract

Instructions:

1. **Prepare the Frozen Yogurt Base:**
   - In a mixing bowl, combine the Greek yogurt, honey or maple syrup, and vanilla extract. Stir well until all ingredients are thoroughly mixed and smooth.
2. **Freeze the Yogurt:**
   - Transfer the yogurt mixture to a freezer-safe container. Cover with a lid or plastic wrap and freeze for about 2-3 hours, stirring every 30 minutes to break up ice crystals and ensure a smooth texture.

- 1 cup fresh fruit, chopped (such as strawberries, blueberries, raspberries, mango, or kiwi)
- Fresh mint leaves (optional, for garnish)

3. **Prepare the Fresh Fruit:**
   - While the yogurt is freezing, wash and chop the fresh fruit into bite-sized pieces. You can use a variety of fruits for a colorful and flavorful combination.
4. **Serve the Frozen Yogurt:**
   - Once the frozen yogurt is firm but scoopable, remove it from the freezer. Scoop the frozen yogurt into bowls.
5. **Top with Fresh Fruit:**
   - Top each serving of frozen yogurt with a generous amount of fresh fruit. Garnish with fresh mint leaves if desired.

Day 16

Breakfast: Banana Nut Muffins

Ingredients:

- 1 1/2 cups whole wheat flour (or a gluten-free flour blend)
- 1 teaspoon baking soda
- 1/2 teaspoon baking powder
- 1/4 teaspoon salt
- 1 teaspoon ground cinnamon
- 1/2 cup walnuts or pecans, chopped
- 3 ripe bananas, mashed

- 1/3 cup honey or maple syrup
- 1/4 cup Greek yogurt (or dairy-free yogurt alternative)
- 1/4 cup olive oil or melted coconut oil
- 1 teaspoon vanilla extract
- 2 large eggs

Instructions:

1. **Preheat the Oven:**
   - Preheat your oven to 350°F (175°C). Line a muffin tin with paper liners or lightly grease it with cooking spray.
2. **Prepare the Dry Ingredients:**
   - In a large mixing bowl, whisk together the whole wheat flour, baking soda, baking powder, salt, and ground cinnamon. Stir in the chopped walnuts or pecans.
3. **Prepare the Wet Ingredients:**
   - In a separate bowl, mash the ripe bananas until smooth. Add the honey or maple syrup, Greek yogurt, olive oil or melted coconut oil, vanilla extract, and eggs. Whisk until all the wet ingredients are well combined.

4. **Combine the Wet and Dry Ingredients:**
   - Pour the wet ingredients into the bowl with the dry ingredients. Stir gently with a spatula or wooden spoon until just combined. Be careful not to overmix; a few lumps are okay.
5. **Fill the Muffin Tin:**
   - Spoon the batter evenly into the prepared muffin tin, filling each cup about 3/4 full.

6. **Bake the Muffins:**
   - Bake in the preheated oven for 18-22 minutes, or until a toothpick inserted into the center of a muffin comes out clean.

7. **Cool the Muffins:**
   - Remove the muffin tin from the oven and let the muffins cool in the tin for 5 minutes. Then, transfer the muffins to a wire rack to cool completely.

Lunch: Grilled Shrimp Tacos with Cabbage Slaw

Ingredients:

For the Grilled Shrimp:

- 1-pound large shrimp, peeled and deveined
- 2 tablespoons olive oil
- 1 teaspoon chili powder
- 1/2 teaspoon cumin
- 1/2 teaspoon paprika
- 1/4 teaspoon garlic powder
- Salt and pepper to taste
- Juice of 1 lime

For the Cabbage Slaw:

- 2 cups shredded green cabbage
- 1 cup shredded red cabbage
- 1/4 cup shredded carrots
- 1/4 cup fresh cilantro, chopped
- 2 tablespoons Greek yogurt or mayonnaise (or dairy-free alternative)
- 1 tablespoon lime juice
- 1 teaspoon honey or maple syrup
- Salt and pepper to taste

For Serving:

- 8 small corn or whole wheat tortillas
- 1 avocado, sliced (optional)
- Lime wedges (optional)
- Hot sauce (optional)

Instructions:

1. **Prepare the Shrimp Marinade:**
   - In a large bowl, combine the olive oil, chili powder, cumin, paprika, garlic powder, salt, pepper, and lime juice. Add the shrimp to the bowl and toss to coat. Let the shrimp marinate for 15-20 minutes while you prepare the slaw.

2. **Prepare the Cabbage Slaw:**
   - In a large mixing bowl, combine the shredded green cabbage, red cabbage, shredded carrots, and chopped cilantro.
   - In a small bowl, whisk together the Greek yogurt or mayonnaise, lime juice, honey or maple syrup, salt, and pepper. Pour the dressing over the

cabbage mixture and toss to combine. Set aside.

3. **Grill the Shrimp:**
   - o Preheat a grill or grill pan over medium-high heat. Thread the shrimp onto skewers (if using a grill) or place them directly onto the grill pan. Grill the shrimp for 2-3 minutes on each side, or until they are pink and opaque. Remove from the grill and set aside.
4. **Warm the Tortillas:**
   - o While the shrimp is grilling, warm the tortillas on the grill or in a dry skillet over medium heat for about 30 seconds on each side, or until soft and pliable.
5. **Assemble the Tacos:**
   - o Place a generous scoop of cabbage slaw onto each tortilla. Top with grilled shrimp and add avocado slices if desired.

Dinner: Chicken Piccata with Zucchini Noodles

Ingredients:

For the Chicken Piccata:

- 2 boneless, skinless chicken breasts, sliced in half lengthwise to create 4 thin cutlets
- Salt and pepper to taste
- 1/4 cup all-purpose flour (or gluten-free flour blend)
- 2 tablespoons olive oil
- 1/4 cup chicken broth (low sodium)
- 1/4 cup fresh lemon juice (about 1-2 lemons)
- 1/4 cup capers, drained and rinsed
- 2 tablespoons unsalted butter
- 2 tablespoons fresh parsley, chopped (optional, for garnish)

For the Zucchini Noodles:

- 3 medium zucchinis, spiralized into noodles (zoodles)
- 1 tablespoon olive oil
- 1 clove garlic, minced
- Salt and pepper to taste
- Red pepper flakes (optional, for a bit of heat)

Instructions:

1. **Prepare the Chicken:**
   - o Season the chicken cutlets with salt and pepper on both sides. Dredge each cutlet in the flour, shaking off any excess.
2. **Cook the Chicken:**
   - o Heat 2 tablespoons of olive oil in a large skillet over medium-high heat. Add the chicken cutlets and cook for about 3-4 minutes on each side, or until golden brown and cooked through. Remove the chicken from the skillet and set aside on a plate.
3. **Make the Piccata Sauce:**
   - o In the same skillet, add the chicken broth, lemon juice, and capers. Bring the mixture to a simmer and cook for about 2-3 minutes, scraping up any browned bits from the bottom of the pan. Stir in the butter until melted and the sauce is slightly thickened.
4. **Return Chicken to the Skillet:**
   - o Return the chicken cutlets to the skillet, spooning the sauce over the top. Simmer for an additional 2 minutes to heat through and allow the flavors to meld. Remove from heat.
5. **Prepare the Zucchini Noodles:**
   - o In a separate skillet, heat 1 tablespoon of olive oil over medium heat. Add the minced garlic and sauté for about 30 seconds until fragrant. Add the spiralized zucchini noodles and sauté for 2-3 minutes, or until the zoodles are just tender but still slightly crisp.

Season with salt, pepper, and red pepper flakes (if using).

6. **Serve the Chicken Piccata with Zoodles:**
    o   Divide the zucchini noodles among serving plates. Place a chicken cutlet on top of each serving of zoodles and spoon the piccata sauce over the chicken.

7. **Garnish and Serve:**
    o   Garnish with fresh parsley if desired.

Snack: Apple Chips

Ingredients:

- 2 large apples (such as Fuji, Honeycrisp, or Granny Smith)
- 1/2 teaspoon ground cinnamon
- 1 tablespoon sugar or honey (optional, for added sweetness)

Instructions:

1. **Preheat the Oven:**
    o   Preheat your oven to 225°F (110°C). Line two baking sheets with parchment paper.

2. **Prepare the Apples:**
    o   Wash and core the apples. Using a sharp knife or a mandolin slicer, slice the apples into thin rings, about 1/8-inch thick. Try to keep the slices as uniform as possible for even baking.

3. **Season the Apple Slices:**
    o   Arrange the apple slices in a single layer on the prepared baking sheets. Sprinkle the apple slices with ground cinnamon and sugar or honey if using.

4. **Bake the Apple Chips:**
    o   Place the baking sheets in the preheated oven. Bake the apple slices for 1 to 1.5 hours, then flip each slice over and continue baking for another 1 to 1.5 hours. The total baking time is about 2 to 3 hours, or until the apples are dry, crispy, and lightly golden. Keep an eye on them to prevent burning.

5. **Cool the Apple Chips:**
    o   Remove the apple chips from the oven and let them cool completely on the baking sheets. They will continue to crisp up as they cool.

6. **Store the Apple Chips:**
    o   Store the cooled apple chips in an airtight container at room temperature for up to a week.

Dessert: Chocolate-Covered Banana Bites

Ingredients:

- 2 ripe bananas
- 1 cup dark chocolate chips or chopped dark chocolate (70% cocoa or higher)
- 1 tablespoon coconut oil
- 1/4 cup chopped nuts (such as almonds, walnuts, or peanuts) or shredded coconut (optional, for topping)
- Sea salt flakes (optional, for garnish)

Instructions:

1. **Prepare the Bananas:**
   - o Peel the bananas and slice them into 1/2-inch-thick rounds. Place the banana slices on a baking sheet lined with parchment paper or a silicone mat.
2. **Freeze the Banana Slices:**
   - o Freeze the banana slices for about 1-2 hours, or until they are firm. This step helps the chocolate coating adhere better to the bananas.
3. **Melt the Chocolate:**
   - o In a microwave-safe bowl, combine the dark chocolate chips and coconut oil. Microwave in 30-second intervals, stirring in between, until the chocolate is completely melted and smooth. Alternatively, you can melt the chocolate in a heatproof bowl set over a pot of simmering water (double boiler method).
4. **Dip the Bananas in Chocolate:**
   - o Using a fork or toothpick, dip each frozen banana slice into the melted chocolate, coating it completely or partially (as you prefer). Let any excess chocolate drip off before placing the dipped banana slice back on the parchment-lined baking sheet.
5. **Add Toppings (Optional):**
   - o While the chocolate is still wet, sprinkle the dipped banana bites with chopped nuts, shredded coconut, or a pinch of sea salt flakes for added flavor and texture.
6. **Freeze the Chocolate-Covered Bananas:**
   - o Return the baking sheet to the freezer and freeze the chocolate-covered banana bites for at least 30 minutes, or until the chocolate is set.
7. **Serve and Enjoy:**
   - o Once the chocolate is fully set, remove the banana bites from the freezer and transfer them to a serving plate.

Day 17

Breakfast: Green Smoothie Bowl with Hemp Seeds

Ingredients:

- 1 cup unsweetened almond milk (or your preferred dairy-free milk)
- 1/2 ripe banana, frozen
- 1/2 cup fresh or frozen mango chunks
- 1 cup fresh spinach leaves
- 1/4 avocado
- 1 tablespoon hemp seeds
- 1 tablespoon honey or maple syrup (optional, for added sweetness)
- A handful of ice cubes (optional, for a thicker smoothie)

Toppings:

- 1 tablespoon hemp seeds
- 1/4 cup fresh berries (such as strawberries, blueberries, or raspberries)
- 1/4 cup granola (choose a low-sugar variety)
- Sliced banana or kiwi (optional)
- A sprinkle of chia seeds or flaxseeds (optional)

Instructions:

1. **Blend the Smoothie:**
   - o In a blender, combine the almond milk, frozen banana, mango chunks, spinach leaves, avocado, hemp seeds, and honey or maple syrup (if using). Add a handful of ice cubes for a thicker, colder texture if desired.
2. **Blend Until Smooth:**

- o Blend on high until all ingredients are fully combined and the smoothie is smooth and creamy.
3. **Prepare the Smoothie Bowl:**
   - o Pour the green smoothie into a bowl.
4. **Add Toppings:**
   - o Top the smoothie bowl with hemp seeds, fresh berries, granola, sliced banana or kiwi, and a sprinkle of chia seeds or flaxseeds for extra nutrition.
5. **Serve and Enjoy:**
   - o Serve immediately and enjoy this refreshing, nutrient-packed breakfast.

Lunch: Roasted Vegetable Wrap with Hummus

Ingredients:

For the Roasted Vegetables:

- 1 medium zucchini, sliced
- 1 red bell pepper, sliced
- 1 yellow bell pepper, sliced
- 1 small red onion, sliced
- 1 tablespoon olive oil
- 1 teaspoon dried oregano
- Salt and pepper to taste

For the Wrap:

- 4 whole wheat or gluten-free tortillas
- 1/2 cup hummus (store-bought or homemade)
- 1/2 cup baby spinach or mixed greens
- 1/4 cup crumbled feta cheese (optional)
- 1/4 cup shredded carrots (optional)
- Fresh herbs (such as basil or parsley, optional, for added flavor)

Instructions:

1. **Preheat the Oven:**
   - o Preheat your oven to 400°F (200°C). Line a baking sheet with parchment paper.
2. **Prepare the Vegetables:**
   - o Place the sliced zucchini, red bell pepper, yellow bell pepper, and red onion on the prepared baking sheet. Drizzle with olive oil and sprinkle with dried oregano, salt, and pepper. Toss to coat the vegetables evenly.
3. **Roast the Vegetables:**
   - o Roast the vegetables in the preheated oven for 15-20 minutes, or until they are tender and slightly caramelized, stirring halfway through to ensure even roasting.
4. **Prepare the Wraps:**
   - o While the vegetables are roasting, warm the tortillas in a dry skillet over medium heat for about 30 seconds on each side, or until soft and pliable.
5. **Assemble the Wraps:**
   - o Spread a generous layer of hummus over each tortilla. Add a handful of baby spinach or mixed greens on top of the hummus.
6. **Add the Roasted Vegetables:**
   - o Once the vegetables are done roasting, divide them evenly among the tortillas, placing them on top of the greens. Sprinkle with crumbled feta cheese and shredded carrots, if using. Add fresh herbs for added flavor if desired.
7. **Roll the Wraps:**
   - o Fold in the sides of each tortilla, then roll it up tightly to enclose the filling.

Dinner: Beef and Veggie Skewers

Ingredients:

For the Skewers:

- 1 pound beef sirloin or tenderloin, cut into 1-inch cubes
- 1 red bell pepper, cut into 1-inch pieces
- 1 yellow bell pepper, cut into 1-inch pieces
- 1 red onion, cut into 1-inch pieces

For the Marinade:

- 3 tablespoons olive oil
- 2 tablespoons soy sauce or tamari (for gluten-free option)
- 2 tablespoons lemon juice
- 2 cloves garlic, minced

- 1 zucchini, sliced into 1/2-inch-thick rounds
- 8-10 cherry tomatoes
- 1 tablespoon olive oil
- Salt and pepper to taste

- 1 teaspoon dried oregano
- 1/2 teaspoon ground black pepper
- 1/2 teaspoon smoked paprika (optional, for added flavor)

Instructions:

1. **Prepare the Marinade:**
   - In a medium bowl, whisk together the olive oil, soy sauce or tamari, lemon juice, minced garlic, dried oregano, black pepper, and smoked paprika (if using).
2. **Marinate the Beef:**
   - Add the beef cubes to the marinade, tossing to coat each piece evenly. Cover and refrigerate for at least 30 minutes, or up to 2 hours for more flavor.
3. **Preheat the Grill:**
   - Preheat your grill or grill pan to medium-high heat.
4. **Prepare the Vegetables:**
   - While the beef is marinating, prepare the vegetables. Cut the bell peppers, red onion, and zucchini into 1-inch pieces. Place the vegetables in a large bowl, drizzle with 1 tablespoon of olive oil, and season with salt and pepper. Toss to coat the vegetables evenly.
5. **Assemble the Skewers:**
   - Thread the marinated beef, bell peppers, red onion, zucchini, and cherry tomatoes onto metal or soaked wooden skewers, alternating between beef and vegetables to create a colorful pattern.
6. **Grill the Skewers:**
   - Place the skewers on the preheated grill. Grill for 8-10 minutes, turning occasionally, until the beef is cooked to your desired level of doneness and the vegetables are tender and slightly charred.
7. **Serve the Skewers:**
   - Remove the skewers from the grill and let them rest for a few minutes. Transfer to a serving platter.

Snack: Greek Yogurt with Chia Seeds

Ingredients:

- 1 cup plain Greek yogurt (or dairy-free yogurt alternative)
- 1 tablespoon chia seeds
- 1-2 teaspoons honey or maple syrup (optional, for added sweetness)
- 1/4 cup fresh berries (such as blueberries, strawberries, or raspberries)
- 1 tablespoon nuts (such as almonds, walnuts, or pecans, chopped)
- A sprinkle of granola (optional, for added crunch)
- A pinch of cinnamon (optional, for extra flavor)

Instructions:

1. **Prepare the Yogurt:**
   - Scoop the Greek yogurt into a serving bowl.
2. **Add Chia Seeds and Sweetener:**
   - Stir in the chia seeds and honey or maple syrup (if using) into the yogurt until well combined. Let it sit for about 5 minutes to allow the chia seeds to absorb some of the moisture and soften slightly.
3. **Add Toppings:**
   - Top the yogurt with fresh berries, chopped nuts, and a sprinkle of granola if desired. Add a pinch of cinnamon for extra flavor if desired.

Dessert: Cinnamon Baked Pears

Ingredients:

- 2 ripe but firm pears (such as Bosc or Anjou)
- 1 tablespoon honey or maple syrup
- 1 teaspoon ground cinnamon
- 1/4 teaspoon ground nutmeg (optional)
- 1/4 cup chopped nuts (such as walnuts, almonds, or pecans)
- 2 tablespoons rolled oats (optional, for added texture)
- 1 tablespoon unsalted butter or coconut oil, melted
- Greek yogurt or whipped cream (optional, for serving)

Instructions:

1. **Preheat the Oven:**
   - Preheat your oven to 350°F (175°C). Lightly grease a baking dish with butter or coconut oil.
2. **Prepare the Pears:**
   - Wash and halve the pears lengthwise. Use a spoon or melon baller to scoop out the core and seeds, creating a small well in the center of each pear half.
3. **Arrange the Pears:**
   - Place the pear halves, cut side up, in the prepared baking dish.
4. **Make the Topping:**
   - In a small bowl, mix together the honey or maple syrup, ground cinnamon, ground nutmeg (if using), chopped

nuts, rolled oats (if using), and melted butter or coconut oil. Stir until the mixture is well combined.

5. **Fill the Pears:**
   - o Spoon the nut and oat mixture into the wells of each pear half, pressing down gently to fill them evenly.

6. **Bake the Pears:**
   - o Bake in the preheated oven for 25-30 minutes, or until the pears are tender and easily pierced with a fork, and the topping is golden and crispy.

7. **Serve the Baked Pears:**
   - o Remove the pears from the oven and let them cool slightly.

8. **Optional Garnishes:**
   - o Serve the baked pears warm, topped with a dollop of Greek yogurt or whipped cream for extra creaminess.

Day 18

Breakfast: Egg and Avocado Breakfast Burrito

Ingredients:

- 4 large eggs
- 1/4 cup milk (dairy or dairy-free alternative)
- Salt and pepper to taste
- 1 tablespoon olive oil or butter
- 1 ripe avocado, sliced
- 1/2 cup cherry tomatoes, halved
- 1/4 cup shredded cheese (such as cheddar or Monterey Jack, optional)
- 2 whole wheat or gluten-free tortillas
- 2 tablespoons fresh cilantro, chopped (optional)
- Hot sauce or salsa (optional, for serving)

Instructions:

1. **Prepare the Eggs:**
   - o In a bowl, whisk together the eggs, milk, salt, and pepper until well combined.
2. **Cook the Eggs:**
   - o Heat the olive oil or butter in a non-stick skillet over medium heat. Pour in the egg mixture and cook, stirring gently, until the eggs are scrambled and just set, about 3-4 minutes. Remove from heat and set aside.
3. **Warm the Tortillas:**
   - o While the eggs are cooking, warm the tortillas in a dry skillet over medium heat for about 30 seconds on each side, or until soft and pliable.
4. **Assemble the Burritos:**
   - o Lay each tortilla flat on a clean surface. Divide the scrambled eggs evenly between the tortillas. Top with sliced avocado, cherry tomatoes, shredded cheese (if using), and chopped cilantro (if desired).
5. **Roll the Burritos:**
   - o Fold in the sides of each tortilla, then roll it up tightly from the bottom to enclose the filling.

Lunch: Asian Chicken Salad with Sesame Dressing

Ingredients:

For the Salad:

- 2 cups cooked chicken breast, shredded or cubed (about 1 large chicken breast)
- 4 cups mixed salad greens (such as romaine, iceberg, or spinach)
- 1 cup shredded red cabbage
- 1/2 cup shredded carrots
- 1/2 red bell pepper, thinly sliced
- 1/2 yellow bell pepper, thinly sliced
- 1/2 cucumber, thinly sliced
- 2 green onions, thinly sliced
- 1/4 cup fresh cilantro, chopped
- 1/4 cup sliced almonds or cashews (optional, for added crunch)
- 1 tablespoon sesame seeds (optional, for garnish)

For the Sesame Dressing:

- 3 tablespoons sesame oil
- 2 tablespoons rice vinegar
- 1 tablespoon soy sauce or tamari (for gluten-free option)
- 1 tablespoon honey or maple syrup
- 1 tablespoon fresh lime juice
- 1 teaspoon grated fresh ginger
- 1 clove garlic, minced
- Salt and pepper to taste

Instructions:

1. **Prepare the Dressing:**
   o In a small bowl, whisk together the sesame oil, rice vinegar, soy sauce or tamari, honey or maple syrup, lime juice, grated ginger, minced garlic, salt, and pepper until well combined. Set aside.
2. **Prepare the Salad Ingredients:**
   o In a large mixing bowl, combine the mixed salad greens, shredded red cabbage, shredded carrots, sliced red and yellow bell peppers, cucumber, green onions, and fresh cilantro.
3. **Add the Chicken:**
   o Add the cooked, shredded or cubed chicken to the bowl with the salad ingredients.
4. **Toss the Salad with Dressing:**
   o Drizzle the sesame dressing over the salad and gently toss to combine all ingredients evenly.
5. **Add Toppings:**
   o Sprinkle the salad with sliced almonds or cashews for added crunch and garnish with sesame seeds if desired.

Dinner: Baked Salmon with Dill Sauce

Ingredients:

For the Baked Salmon:

- 4 salmon fillets (about 6 ounces each)
- 1 tablespoon olive oil
- Salt and pepper to taste
- 1 lemon, thinly sliced
- Fresh dill sprigs (optional, for garnish)

For the Dill Sauce:

- 1/2 cup Greek yogurt (or dairy-free yogurt alternative)
- 1 tablespoon mayonnaise (optional, for creaminess)
- 1 tablespoon fresh lemon juice
- 1 tablespoon fresh dill, chopped
- 1 teaspoon Dijon mustard
- 1 clove garlic, minced
- Salt and pepper to taste

Instructions:

1. **Preheat the Oven:**
   - o Preheat your oven to 375°F (190°C). Line a baking sheet with parchment paper or lightly grease it with olive oil.

2. **Prepare the Salmon:**
   - o Place the salmon fillets on the prepared baking sheet, skin side down. Drizzle with olive oil and season with salt and pepper. Arrange lemon slices on top of each fillet.

3. **Bake the Salmon:**
   - o Bake the salmon in the preheated oven for 12-15 minutes, or until the salmon is opaque and flakes easily with a fork. Cooking time may vary depending on the thickness of the fillets.

4. **Prepare the Dill Sauce:**
   - o While the salmon is baking, prepare the dill sauce. In a small bowl, combine the Greek yogurt, mayonnaise (if using), lemon juice, chopped fresh dill, Dijon mustard, minced garlic, salt, and pepper. Stir until well combined. Adjust seasoning to taste.

5. **Serve the Salmon:**
   - o Once the salmon is done baking, remove it from the oven. Transfer the fillets to serving plates.

6. **Add the Dill Sauce:**
   - o Spoon the dill sauce over the baked salmon fillets or serve it on the side.

7. **Garnish and Serve:**
   - o Garnish with fresh dill sprigs and extra lemon slices if desired.

Snack: Carrot and Celery Sticks with Guacamole

Ingredients:

For the Guacamole:

- 2 ripe avocados
- 1/4 cup red onion, finely diced
- 1 small tomato, diced
- 1 clove garlic, minced
- 1 tablespoon fresh lime juice
- 2 tablespoons fresh cilantro, chopped
- Salt and pepper to taste
- A pinch of cayenne pepper (optional, for a bit of heat)

For the Veggie Sticks:

- 2 large carrots, peeled and cut into sticks
- 3-4 celery stalks, cut into sticks

- **Instructions:**

1. **Prepare the Guacamole:**
   - o Cut the avocados in half, remove the pits, and scoop the flesh into a medium bowl. Mash the avocado with a fork or potato masher until it reaches your desired consistency (smooth or chunky).
   - o Add the diced red onion, diced tomato, minced garlic, lime juice, and chopped cilantro to the mashed avocado. Mix well to combine.
   - o Season the guacamole with salt, pepper, and cayenne pepper (if using) to taste. Stir to incorporate all the flavors.

2. **Prepare the Veggie Sticks:**
   - o Wash, peel, and cut the carrots into sticks. Wash and cut the celery stalks into sticks. Arrange them on a serving platter.

3. **Serve the Guacamole with Veggie Sticks:**
   - o Transfer the guacamole to a small bowl and place it in the center of the serving

platter with the carrot and celery sticks
arranged around it

Dessert: Key Lime Pie

Ingredients:

For the Crust:

- 1 1/2 cups graham cracker crumbs (or gluten-free graham crackers, crushed)
- 1/4 cup granulated sugar
- 6 tablespoons unsalted butter, melted

For the Filling:

- 1 can (14 ounces) sweetened condensed milk
- 1/2 cup Greek yogurt (or dairy-free yogurt alternative)
- 1/2 cup fresh key lime juice (about 4-5 key limes)
- 1 tablespoon lime zest
- 3 large egg yolks

For the Topping:

- 1 cup heavy whipping cream (or coconut cream for a dairy-free option)
- 2 tablespoons powdered sugar
- 1/2 teaspoon vanilla extract
- Lime slices or zest (optional, for garnish)

Instructions:

1. **Preheat the Oven:**
   - Preheat your oven to 350°F (175°C).
2. **Prepare the Crust:**
   - In a medium mixing bowl, combine the graham cracker crumbs, granulated sugar, and melted butter. Stir until the mixture resembles wet sand.
   - Press the crumb mixture evenly into the bottom and up the sides of a 9-inch pie dish. Use the bottom of a measuring cup or glass to press the crust firmly into place.
   - Bake the crust in the preheated oven for 8-10 minutes, or until lightly golden. Remove from the oven and let it cool slightly.
3. **Make the Filling:**
   - In a large mixing bowl, whisk together the sweetened condensed milk, Greek yogurt, key lime juice, lime zest, and egg yolks until smooth and well combined.
4. **Fill the Crust:**
   - Pour the filling into the slightly cooled graham cracker crust and spread it out evenly.
5. **Bake the Pie:**
   - Bake the pie in the preheated oven for 15-20 minutes, or until the filling is set but still slightly jiggly in the center.
6. **Cool and Chill the Pie:**
   - Remove the pie from the oven and let it cool to room temperature. Once cooled, refrigerate the pie for at least 2 hours, or until fully chilled and set.
7. **Prepare the Whipped Cream Topping:**
   - In a medium mixing bowl, beat the heavy whipping cream, powdered sugar, and vanilla extract with an electric mixer on medium-high speed until soft peaks form.
8. **Top the Pie:**
   - Spread or pipe the whipped cream over the chilled pie. Garnish with lime slices or additional lime zest if desired.

Day 19

Breakfast: Peanut Butter Banana Smoothie

Ingredients:

- 1 ripe banana, frozen
- 1 tablespoon peanut butter (unsweetened and natural)
- 1/2 cup Greek yogurt (or dairy-free yogurt alternative)
- 1 cup unsweetened almond milk (or your preferred dairy-free milk)
- 1 tablespoon honey or maple syrup (optional, for added sweetness)
- 1/2 teaspoon vanilla extract (optional)
- A handful of ice cubes (optional, for a thicker, colder smoothie)
- 1 tablespoon chia seeds or flaxseeds (optional, for added fiber and nutrition)

Instructions:

1. **Prepare the Ingredients:**
   - Peel and slice the banana and freeze it ahead of time for a thicker, creamier smoothie.
2. **Blend the Smoothie:**
   - In a blender, combine the frozen banana, peanut butter, Greek yogurt, almond milk, honey or maple syrup (if using), vanilla extract (if using), and chia seeds or flaxseeds (if using).
3. **Add Ice and Blend Until Smooth:**
   - If you prefer a thicker, colder smoothie, add a handful of ice cubes. Blend on high until all the ingredients are fully combined and the smoothie is smooth and creamy.

Lunch: Chickpea and Tomato Salad

Ingredients:

- 1 can (15 ounces) chickpeas, drained and rinsed
- 1 cup cherry tomatoes, halved
- 1/2 cucumber, diced
- 1/4 red onion, finely chopped
- 1/4 cup Kalamata olives, pitted and sliced (optional)
- 1/4 cup feta cheese, crumbled (optional)
- 2 tablespoons fresh parsley, chopped
- 2 tablespoons fresh basil, chopped (optional)
- 1 tablespoon capers, drained (optional)

For the Dressing:

- 3 tablespoons extra-virgin olive oil
- 2 tablespoons red wine vinegar
- 1 tablespoon fresh lemon juice
- 1 teaspoon Dijon mustard
- 1 clove garlic, minced
- Salt and pepper to taste

Instructions:

1. **Prepare the Salad Ingredients:**
   - o   In a large mixing bowl, combine the drained and rinsed chickpeas, halved cherry tomatoes, diced cucumber, finely chopped red onion, sliced Kalamata olives (if using), crumbled feta cheese (if using), chopped parsley, basil (if using), and capers (if using).
2. **Make the Dressing:**
   - o   In a small bowl, whisk together the extra-virgin olive oil, red wine vinegar, lemon juice, Dijon mustard, minced garlic, salt, and pepper until well combined.
3. **Toss the Salad with Dressing:**
   - o   Pour the dressing over the chickpea and vegetable mixture. Toss gently to combine all the ingredients evenly and ensure they are well coated with the dressing.
4. **Serve the Salad:**
   - o   Divide the chickpea and tomato salad into serving bowls or plates.

Dinner: Turkey Meatballs with Marinara and Spaghetti Squash

Ingredients:

For the Turkey Meatballs:

- 1 pound ground turkey
- 1/4 cup breadcrumbs (whole wheat or gluten-free)
- 1/4 cup grated Parmesan cheese (optional)
- 1/4 cup fresh parsley, chopped
- 1 egg, beaten
- 2 cloves garlic, minced
- 1 teaspoon dried oregano
- 1/2 teaspoon salt
- 1/4 teaspoon black pepper
- 1 tablespoon olive oil (for cooking)

For the Marinara Sauce:

- 1 tablespoon olive oil
- 1 small onion, finely chopped
- 2 cloves garlic, minced
- 1 can (28 ounces) crushed tomatoes
- 1 teaspoon dried basil
- 1 teaspoon dried oregano
- Salt and pepper to taste
- A pinch of red pepper flakes (optional, for a bit of heat)

For the Spaghetti Squash:

- 1 medium spaghetti squash
- 1 tablespoon olive oil
- Salt and pepper to taste

Instructions:

1. **Prepare the Spaghetti Squash:**
   - o   Preheat your oven to 400°F (200°C). Line a baking sheet with parchment paper.
   - o   Cut the spaghetti squash in half lengthwise and scoop out the seeds with a spoon.
   - o   Drizzle the cut sides with olive oil and season with salt and pepper. Place the

squash halves cut side down on the prepared baking sheet and roast for 35-40 minutes, or until the squash is tender and can be easily shredded with a fork.

2. **Make the Turkey Meatballs:**
   o In a large mixing bowl, combine the ground turkey, breadcrumbs, Parmesan cheese (if using), chopped parsley, beaten egg, minced garlic, dried oregano, salt, and pepper. Mix until all ingredients are well combined.
   o Form the mixture into small meatballs, about 1 inch in diameter.
   o Heat 1 tablespoon of olive oil in a large skillet over medium heat. Add the meatballs in a single layer and cook for 8-10 minutes, turning occasionally, until they are browned on all sides and cooked through. Remove the meatballs from the skillet and set aside.

3. **Prepare the Marinara Sauce:**
   o In the same skillet, heat 1 tablespoon of olive oil over medium heat. Add the chopped onion and sauté for 3-4 minutes, until softened. Add the minced garlic and sauté for another 1 minute until fragrant.
   o Pour in the crushed tomatoes, dried basil, dried oregano, salt, pepper, and red pepper flakes (if using). Stir to combine and bring the sauce to a simmer. Let it cook for 10-15 minutes, stirring occasionally, until the sauce thickens slightly.

4. **Combine Meatballs with Marinara:**
   o Add the cooked turkey meatballs to the marinara sauce, gently stirring to coat them with the sauce. Simmer for an additional 5 minutes to allow the flavors to meld.

5. **Prepare the Spaghetti Squash:**
   o Once the spaghetti squash is roasted, remove it from the oven and let it cool slightly. Use a fork to scrape the inside of each squash half to create spaghetti-like strands.

6. **Serve the Dish:**
   o Divide the spaghetti squash strands among serving plates. Top with turkey meatballs and marinara sauce.

7. **Garnish and Serve:**
   o Garnish with additional chopped parsley and grated Parmesan cheese if desired.

Snack: Almonds and Walnuts

Ingredients:

- 1/4 cup raw or roasted almonds
- 1/4 cup raw or roasted walnuts

Instructions:

1. **Prepare the Nuts:**
   o If using raw nuts, you can choose to roast them for added flavor. Preheat your oven to 350°F (175°C). Spread the almonds and walnuts on a baking sheet in a single layer and roast for 8-10 minutes, stirring halfway through, until they are golden and fragrant. Let them cool completely.

2. **Mix the Nuts:**
   o Combine the almonds and walnuts in a small bowl or resealable snack bag.

3. **Serve and Enjoy:**
   o Enjoy this simple and nutritious snack any time you need a quick energy boost.

Dessert: Strawberry Shortcake

Ingredients:

For the Shortcakes:

- 2 cups all-purpose flour (or a gluten-free flour blend)
- 1/4 cup granulated sugar
- 1 tablespoon baking powder
- 1/2 teaspoon salt
- 1/2 cup cold unsalted butter, cut into small cubes
- 3/4 cup milk (dairy or dairy-free alternative)
- 1 large egg, beaten
- 1 teaspoon vanilla extract

For the Strawberry Topping:

- 2 cups fresh strawberries, hulled and sliced
- 2 tablespoons granulated sugar
- 1 tablespoon fresh lemon juice

For the Whipped Cream:

- 1 cup heavy whipping cream (or coconut cream for a dairy-free option)
- 2 tablespoons powdered sugar
- 1/2 teaspoon vanilla extract

Instructions:

1. **Prepare the Strawberries:**
   - In a medium bowl, combine the sliced strawberries, granulated sugar, and lemon juice. Stir well and let the mixture sit at room temperature for at least 30 minutes to macerate, allowing the strawberries to release their juices.
2. **Preheat the Oven:**
   - Preheat your oven to 425°F (220°C). Line a baking sheet with parchment paper.
3. **Make the Shortcakes:**
   - In a large mixing bowl, whisk together the flour, sugar, baking powder, and salt. Add the cold butter cubes and use a pastry cutter or your fingers to cut the butter into the flour mixture until it resembles coarse crumbs.
   - In a separate bowl, whisk together the milk, beaten egg, and vanilla extract. Pour the wet ingredients into the dry ingredients and stir until just combined. Do not overmix; the dough should be slightly sticky.
   - Turn the dough out onto a lightly floured surface and gently knead it a few times to bring it together. Pat the dough into a 1-inch-thick circle. Use a biscuit cutter or a glass to cut out 8 shortcakes, re-rolling the dough scraps as needed.
4. **Bake the Shortcakes:**
   - Place the shortcakes on the prepared baking sheet and brush the tops with a little milk or egg wash for a golden finish. Bake in the preheated oven for 12-15 minutes, or until the shortcakes are golden brown and cooked through. Remove from the oven and let them cool on a wire rack.
5. **Prepare the Whipped Cream:**
   - In a medium mixing bowl, beat the heavy whipping cream, powdered sugar, and vanilla extract with an electric mixer on medium-high speed until soft peaks form. If using coconut cream, make sure it's well-chilled and only use the solid part; beat as you would heavy cream.
6. **Assemble the Strawberry Shortcakes:**

o Once the shortcakes are cool, split them in half horizontally with a serrated knife. Place the bottom halves on serving plates, spoon a generous number of macerated strawberries and their juices over each, then top with a dollop of whipped cream. Place the top halves of the shortcakes over the whipped cream.

Day 20

Breakfast: Savory Quinoa Breakfast Bowl

Ingredients:

- 1/2 cup quinoa, rinsed
- 1 cup water or low-sodium vegetable broth
- 1 tablespoon olive oil
- 2 large eggs
- 1/2 avocado, sliced
- 1/2 cup cherry tomatoes, halved
- 1/4 cup cucumber, diced
- 1/4 cup feta cheese, crumbled (optional)
- 2 tablespoons fresh parsley or cilantro, chopped
- Salt and pepper to taste
- Hot sauce or salsa (optional, for serving)
- 1 tablespoon lemon juice (optional, for added flavor)

Instructions:

1. **Cook the Quinoa:**
   - o In a medium saucepan, bring the water or vegetable broth to a boil. Add the rinsed quinoa, reduce the heat to low, cover, and simmer for about 15 minutes, or until the quinoa is tender and the liquid is absorbed. Remove from heat and let it sit, covered, for 5 minutes. Fluff with a fork and set aside.
2. **Prepare the Eggs:**
   - o While the quinoa is cooking, heat 1 tablespoon of olive oil in a non-stick skillet over medium heat. Crack the eggs into the skillet and cook to your desired level of doneness (sunny side up, over easy, or scrambled). Season with salt and pepper to taste. Remove from heat and set aside.
3. **Assemble the Breakfast Bowl:**
   - o Divide the cooked quinoa between two bowls. Arrange the avocado slices, cherry tomatoes, cucumber, and cooked eggs on top of the quinoa in each bowl.
4. **Add Toppings:**
   - o Sprinkle with crumbled feta cheese (if using) and chopped fresh parsley or cilantro. Drizzle with lemon juice for added flavor, if desired.

Lunch: Greek Salad with Grilled Chicken

Ingredients:

For the Grilled Chicken:

- 2 boneless, skinless chicken breasts
- 1 tablespoon olive oil
- 1 tablespoon lemon juice
- 1 teaspoon dried oregano
- 1/2 teaspoon garlic powder
- Salt and pepper to taste

For the Greek Salad:

- 4 cups romaine lettuce, chopped
- 1 cup cherry tomatoes, halved
- 1/2 cucumber, sliced
- 1/4 red onion, thinly sliced
- 1/2 cup Kalamata olives, pitted and halved

For the Dressing:

- 3 tablespoons extra-virgin olive oil
- 2 tablespoons red wine vinegar
- 1 teaspoon Dijon mustard
- 1 teaspoon dried oregano

Instructions:

- 1/2 cup feta cheese, crumbled (optional)
- 1/4 cup red or green bell pepper, sliced
- 2 tablespoons fresh parsley, chopped (optional)

- 1 clove garlic, minced
- Salt and pepper to taste

1. **Marinate the Chicken:**
   - In a small bowl, combine the olive oil, lemon juice, dried oregano, garlic powder, salt, and pepper. Place the chicken breasts in a shallow dish or a resealable plastic bag, and pour the marinade over the chicken. Let it marinate for at least 15 minutes (or up to 1 hour) in the refrigerator.
2. **Grill the Chicken:**
   - Preheat a grill or grill pan over medium-high heat. Remove the chicken from the marinade and grill for about 5-7 minutes on each side, or until the chicken is cooked through and has reached an internal temperature of 165°F (75°C). Remove from the grill and let the chicken rest for a few minutes before slicing it into thin strips.
3. **Prepare the Dressing:**
   - In a small bowl, whisk together the olive oil, red wine vinegar, Dijon mustard, dried oregano, minced garlic, salt, and pepper until well combined.
4. **Assemble the Salad:**
   - In a large mixing bowl, combine the chopped romaine lettuce, cherry tomatoes, cucumber slices, red onion, Kalamata olives, bell pepper slices, and crumbled feta cheese (if using).
5. **Add the Grilled Chicken:**
   - Top the salad with the sliced grilled chicken.
6. **Dress the Salad:**
   - Drizzle the dressing over the salad and toss gently to combine all the ingredients and coat them evenly with the dressing.
7. **Serve and Enjoy:**
   - Divide the Greek salad with grilled chicken into serving plates. Garnish with fresh parsley if desired.

Dinner: Miso-Glazed Cod with Bok Choy

Ingredients:

For the Miso-Glazed Cod:

- 4 cod fillets (about 6 ounces each)
- 2 tablespoons white miso paste
- 1 tablespoon mirin (sweet rice wine)
- 1 tablespoon soy sauce or tamari (for gluten-free option)

- 1 tablespoon honey or maple syrup
- 1 tablespoon rice vinegar
- 1 teaspoon sesame oil
- 1 clove garlic, minced
- 1 teaspoon fresh ginger, grated

For the Bok Choy:

- 4 baby Bok choy, halved lengthwise
- 1 tablespoon olive oil or sesame oil
- 2 cloves garlic, minced
- 1 teaspoon fresh ginger, grated

- 2 tablespoons low-sodium soy sauce or tamari
- 1 tablespoon rice vinegar
- 1 teaspoon sesame seeds (optional, for garnish)

Instructions:

1. **Prepare the Miso Glaze:**
   - In a small bowl, whisk together the white miso paste, mirin, soy sauce or tamari, honey or maple syrup, rice vinegar, sesame oil, minced garlic, and grated ginger until smooth and well combined.
2. **Marinate the Cod:**
   - Place the cod fillets in a shallow dish or resealable plastic bag. Pour the miso glaze over the cod, ensuring each fillet is well coated. Marinate in the refrigerator for at least 30 minutes, or up to 1 hour for more flavor.
3. **Preheat the Oven:**
   - Preheat your oven to 400°F (200°C). Line a baking sheet with parchment paper or lightly grease it with oil.
4. **Bake the Cod:**
   - Remove the cod from the marinade and place the fillets on the prepared baking sheet. Bake in the preheated oven for 10-12 minutes, or until the cod is opaque and flakes easily with a fork.
5. **Prepare the Bok Choy:**
   - While the cod is baking, heat the olive oil or sesame oil in a large skillet or wok over medium-high heat. Add the minced garlic and grated ginger, and sauté for about 30 seconds until fragrant.
   - Add the halved Bok choy to the skillet and cook for 3-4 minutes, stirring occasionally, until the Bok choy is tender but still crisp.
6. **Add the Sauce:**
   - In a small bowl, whisk together the soy sauce or tamari and rice vinegar. Pour the sauce over the Bok choy in the skillet and toss to coat. Cook for an additional 1-2 minutes until the Bok choy is fully coated and the sauce is heated through.
7. **Serve the Dish:**
   - Divide the miso-glazed cod fillets and Bok choy among serving plates.

Snack: Seaweed Snacks

Ingredients:

- 1 package of dried seaweed sheets (nori), typically used for sushi
- 1 teaspoon sesame oil (optional, for flavor)

- A pinch of sea salt or seasoning blend (optional, for added flavor)
- 1/2 teaspoon sesame seeds (optional, for garnish)

Instructions:

1. **Prepare the Seaweed Sheets:**
   - If your seaweed sheets are not already pre-cut, use kitchen scissors to cut them into snack-sized pieces (about 2x2 inches).
2. **Add Flavor (Optional):**
   - If you prefer your seaweed snacks with a little extra flavor, lightly brush each seaweed sheet with sesame oil using a pastry brush. Sprinkle a pinch of sea salt or your favorite seasoning blend on top for added taste. You can also

sprinkle sesame seeds on top for a bit of crunch and nutty flavor.

3. **Serve and Enjoy:**
   - Place the seaweed sheets on a serving plate. They are ready to eat as is, no additional preparation needed.

4. **Store Leftovers:**
   - Store any leftover seaweed snacks in an airtight container at room temperature to maintain crispness.

Dessert: Berry Crumble

Ingredients:

For the Berry Filling:

- 4 cups mixed fresh berries (such as strawberries, blueberries, raspberries, and blackberries)
- 2 tablespoons granulated sugar or honey (adjust to taste)
- 1 tablespoon lemon juice
- 1 tablespoon cornstarch or arrowroot powder

For the Crumble Topping:

- 1 cup rolled oats (use gluten-free oats if needed)
- 1/2 cup almond flour (or regular flour)
- 1/4 cup brown sugar or coconut sugar
- 1/2 teaspoon ground cinnamon
- 1/4 teaspoon salt
- 1/4 cup unsalted butter or coconut oil, melted
- 1/4 cup chopped nuts (such as almonds or pecans, optional)

Instructions:

1. **Preheat the Oven:**
   - Preheat your oven to 350°F (175°C). Grease a 9-inch baking dish with butter or coconut oil.

2. **Prepare the Berry Filling:**
   - In a large bowl, combine the mixed berries, granulated sugar or honey, lemon juice, and cornstarch or arrowroot powder. Toss gently to coat the berries evenly. Pour the berry mixture into the prepared baking dish.

3. **Make the Crumble Topping:**
   - In a medium bowl, combine the rolled oats, almond flour, brown sugar or coconut sugar, ground cinnamon, and salt. Add the melted butter or coconut oil and mix until the mixture is crumbly and well combined. Stir in the chopped nuts, if using.

4. **Assemble the Crumble:**
   - Sprinkle the crumble topping evenly over the berry filling in the baking dish.

5. **Bake the Crumble:**
   - Bake in the preheated oven for 30-35 minutes, or until the topping is golden brown and the berry filling is bubbling.

6. **Cool and Serve:**
   - Remove the berry crumble from the oven and let it cool for a few minutes. Serve warm.

7. **Optional Garnish:**
   - Serve the berry crumble with a scoop of vanilla ice cream, a dollop of Greek yogurt, or a drizzle of honey for added sweetness.

Day 21

Breakfast: Cottage Cheese with Fresh Fruit

Ingredients:

- 1 cup cottage cheese (low-fat or full fat, depending on preference)
- 1/2 cup fresh fruit, diced (such as strawberries, blueberries, raspberries, kiwi, or peaches)
- 1 tablespoon honey or maple syrup (optional, for added sweetness)
- 1 tablespoon chopped nuts (such as almonds, walnuts, or pecans, optional)
- A sprinkle of cinnamon (optional, for extra flavor)
- Fresh mint leaves (optional, for garnish)

Instructions:

1. **Prepare the Cottage Cheese:**
   o Scoop the cottage cheese into a serving bowl.
2. **Add the Fresh Fruit:**
   o Top the cottage cheese with your choice of fresh, diced fruit. You can mix and match different fruits for a colorful and flavorful combination.
3. **Optional Sweetener:**
   o Drizzle honey or maple syrup over the fruit and cottage cheese if you prefer a sweeter taste.
4. **Add Toppings:**
   o Sprinkle chopped nuts over the top for added crunch and healthy fats. Add a sprinkle of cinnamon for extra flavor, if desired.
5. **Garnish and Serve:**
   o Garnish with fresh mint leaves for a touch of color and freshness, if desired.

Lunch: Avocado and Tomato Salad with Lime Dressing

Ingredients:

For the Salad:

- 2 ripe avocados, diced
- 1 1/2 cups cherry tomatoes, halved
- 1/2 red onion, finely chopped
- 1/2 cucumber, diced
- 1/4 cup fresh cilantro, chopped (optional)
- 1/4 cup feta cheese, crumbled (optional)
- 1/4 cup corn kernels (fresh, canned, or frozen, optional)

For the Lime Dressing:

- 3 tablespoons extra-virgin olive oil
- 2 tablespoons fresh lime juice (about 1 lime)
- 1 teaspoon honey or agave syrup (optional, for sweetness)
- 1 clove garlic, minced
- Salt and pepper to taste
- 1/2 teaspoon ground cumin (optional, for added flavor)

1. **Prepare the Salad Ingredients:**
    o In a large mixing bowl, combine the diced avocados, halved cherry tomatoes, chopped red onion, diced cucumber, fresh cilantro, feta cheese (if using), and corn kernels (if using).
2. **Make the Lime Dressing:**
    o In a small bowl, whisk together the extra-virgin olive oil, fresh lime juice, honey or agave syrup (if using), minced garlic, salt, pepper, and ground cumin (if using) until well combined.
3. **Toss the Salad with Dressing:**
    o Pour the lime dressing over the salad ingredients in the bowl. Gently toss to combine, ensuring all ingredients are evenly coated with the dressing.
4. **Serve the Salad:**
    o Divide the avocado and tomato salad into serving bowls or plates.

Dinner: Thai Peanut Chicken with Brown Rice

Ingredients:

For the Thai Peanut Chicken:

- 1-pound boneless, skinless chicken breast, cut into bite-sized pieces
- 1 tablespoon olive oil
- 1 red bell pepper, sliced
- 1 cup snap peas or green beans, trimmed
- 2 cloves garlic, minced
- 1 tablespoon fresh ginger, grated
- 1/4 cup green onions, sliced (optional, for garnish)
- 2 tablespoons fresh cilantro, chopped (optional, for garnish)
- 1/4 cup chopped peanuts (optional, for garnish)

For the Peanut Sauce:

- 1/3 cup creamy peanut butter
- 2 tablespoons soy sauce or tamari (for gluten-free option)
- 1 tablespoon rice vinegar
- 1 tablespoon honey or maple syrup
- 1 tablespoon fresh lime juice (about 1 lime)
- 1 teaspoon sesame oil
- 1/2 teaspoon red pepper flakes (optional, for a bit of heat)
- 1/4 cup water (to thin the sauce, if needed)

For the Brown Rice:

- 1 cup brown rice
- 2 cups water or low-sodium chicken broth
- 1/4 teaspoon salt

Instructions:

1. **Cook the Brown Rice:**
    o In a medium saucepan, combine the brown rice, water or chicken broth, and salt. Bring to a boil, then reduce the heat to low, cover, and simmer for about 40-45 minutes, or until the rice is tender and the liquid is absorbed. Remove from heat and let it sit,

covered, for 5 minutes. Fluff with a fork and set aside.

2. **Prepare the Peanut Sauce:**
   - In a small bowl, whisk together the peanut butter, soy sauce or tamari, rice vinegar, honey or maple syrup, lime juice, sesame oil, red pepper flakes (if using), and water. Adjust the consistency with more water if needed, to reach a smooth, pourable sauce. Set aside.

3. **Cook the Chicken and Vegetables:**
   - Heat the olive oil in a large skillet or wok over medium-high heat. Add the chicken pieces and cook for 5-7 minutes, stirring occasionally, until the chicken is browned and cooked through.
   - Add the minced garlic and grated ginger to the skillet and sauté for 1 minute until fragrant.
   - Add the sliced red bell pepper and snap peas or green beans. Cook for an additional 3-4 minutes, or until the vegetables are tender-crisp.

4. **Add the Peanut Sauce:**
   - Pour the peanut sauce over the chicken and vegetables in the skillet. Stir to coat everything evenly and cook for another 2-3 minutes, until the sauce is heated through and slightly thickened.

5. **Serve the Dish:**
   - Divide the cooked brown rice among serving plates. Top with the Thai peanut chicken and vegetables.

6. **Garnish and Serve:**
   - Garnish with sliced green onions, fresh cilantro, and chopped peanuts, if desired.

Snack: Zucchini Chips

Ingredients:

- 2 medium zucchinis
- 1 tablespoon olive oil
- 1/2 teaspoon sea salt
- 1/2 teaspoon garlic powder (optional, for added flavor)
- 1/4 teaspoon paprika (optional, for added flavor)
- A pinch of black pepper (optional)

Instructions:

1. **Preheat the Oven:**
   - Preheat your oven to 225°F (110°C). Line a baking sheet with parchment paper or a silicone baking mat.

2. **Prepare the Zucchini:**
   - Wash and dry the zucchinis. Using a sharp knife or a mandolin slicer, slice the zucchinis into very thin rounds, about 1/8-inch thick. Try to keep the slices as uniform as possible for even baking.

3. **Season the Zucchini:**
   - In a large mixing bowl, toss the zucchini slices with olive oil until they are evenly coated. Sprinkle the sea salt, garlic powder, paprika, and black pepper over the zucchini slices and toss again to coat evenly.

4. **Arrange the Zucchini on the Baking Sheet:**
   - Arrange the zucchini slices in a single layer on the prepared baking sheet. Make sure the slices are not overlapping to ensure they bake evenly.

5. **Bake the Zucchini Chips:**
   - Bake in the preheated oven for 1.5 to 2 hours, or until the zucchini slices are crispy and golden brown. Check the chips occasionally to ensure they are not burning and rotate the baking sheet if necessary for even baking.

6. **Cool and Serve:**
   - Remove the zucchini chips from the oven and let them cool on the baking sheet for a few minutes. They will continue to crisp up as they cool.

7. **Store Leftovers:**

     o   Store any leftover zucchini chips in an airtight container at room temperature for up to 3 days to maintain their crispness.

Dessert: Cherry Chocolate Chip Ice Cream

Ingredients:

- 1/2 cup dark chocolate chips or chopped dark chocolate (70% cocoa or higher) 2 cups fresh or frozen cherries, pitted
- 1 cup heavy cream (or coconut cream for a dairy-free option)
- 1 cup whole milk (or almond milk for a dairy-free option)
- 1/2 cup granulated sugar or honey (adjust to taste)
- 1 teaspoon vanilla extract

Instructions:

1. **Prepare the Cherry Mixture:**
   - In a blender or food processor, blend the pitted cherries until smooth. If you prefer chunks of cherries in your ice cream, blend only half of the cherries until smooth and chop the remaining cherries into small pieces. Set aside.
2. **Make the Ice Cream Base:**
   - In a medium mixing bowl, whisk together the heavy cream, whole milk, sugar or honey, and vanilla extract until the sugar is completely dissolved.
3. **Combine the Cherry Mixture and Ice Cream Base:**
   - Stir the blended cherry mixture into the ice cream base. Mix until well combined.
4. **Churn the Ice Cream:**
   - Pour the mixture into an ice cream maker and churn according to the manufacturer's instructions, usually about 20-25 minutes, or until the ice cream reaches a soft-serve consistency.
5. **Add the Chocolate Chips:**
   - During the last 5 minutes of churning, add the dark chocolate chips or chopped chocolate to the ice cream maker and let it mix until evenly distributed.
6. **Freeze the Ice Cream:**
   - Transfer the churned ice cream to an airtight container. Cover and freeze for at least 2-4 hours, or until the ice cream is firm.

Week 4: Mastering Your Diet

Day 22

Breakfast: Baked Eggs in Avocado

Ingredients:

- 2 ripe avocados, halved and pitted
- 4 large eggs
- Salt and pepper to taste

Instructions:

- 1/4 teaspoon paprika or chili powder (optional, for added flavor)
- Fresh herbs, such as chives, parsley, or cilantro, chopped (optional, for garnish)
- Hot sauce or salsa (optional, for serving)

1. **Preheat the Oven:**
   o Preheat your oven to 375°F (190°C). Line a baking sheet with parchment paper or lightly grease it with cooking spray.
2. **Prepare the Avocados:**
   o Cut the avocados in half and remove the pits. If needed, scoop out a small amount of the flesh to create a larger well that can hold the egg.

3. **Prepare the Eggs:**
   o Carefully crack an egg into each avocado half, letting the yolk settle into the well where the pit was. The egg whites may overflow slightly,

depending on the size of the avocados. Season the eggs with salt, pepper, and paprika or chili powder (if using).

4. **Bake the Avocados:**
   o Place the avocado halves on the prepared baking sheet. Bake in the preheated oven for 15-20 minutes, or until the egg whites are set and the yolks are cooked to your desired level of doneness.
5. **Garnish and Serve:**
   o Remove the baked eggs in avocado from the oven and let them cool slightly. Garnish with fresh herbs if desired and add a few dashes of hot sauce or a spoonful of salsa for extra flavor.

Lunch: Salmon and Avocado Rice Bowl

Ingredients:

- 1 cup cooked brown rice or white rice
- 4 ounces cooked salmon (grilled, baked, or poached)
- 1/2 avocado, sliced
- 1/2 cucumber, thinly sliced
- 1/2 cup shredded carrots
- 1/4 cup edamame (shelled and cooked)
- 1 tablespoon sesame seeds (optional, for garnish)
- 2 tablespoons green onions, sliced (optional, for garnish)
- Fresh cilantro or parsley, chopped (optional, for garnish)

For the Dressing:

- 2 tablespoons soy sauce or tamari (for gluten-free option)
- 1 tablespoon rice vinegar
- 1 tablespoon sesame oil
- 1 teaspoon honey or maple syrup
- 1 teaspoon fresh ginger, grated
- 1 clove garlic, minced

Instructions:

1. **Prepare the Dressing:**
   - o   In a small bowl, whisk together the soy sauce or tamari, rice vinegar, sesame oil, honey or maple syrup, grated ginger, and minced garlic until well combined. Set aside.
2. **Assemble the Rice Bowl:**
   - o   Divide the cooked brown rice into two serving bowls.
3. **Add the Toppings:**
   - o   Top each bowl of rice with flaked salmon, sliced avocado, cucumber, shredded carrots, and edamame.
4. **Drizzle with Dressing:**
   - o   Drizzle the prepared dressing evenly over each bowl.
5. **Garnish the Bowls:**
   - o   Sprinkle with sesame seeds, sliced green onions, and chopped cilantro or parsley if desired.

Dinner: Moroccan Chicken with Couscous

Ingredients:

For the Moroccan Chicken:

- 1-pound boneless, skinless chicken thighs or breasts, cut into bite-sized pieces
- 1 tablespoon olive oil
- 1 medium onion, finely chopped
- 2 cloves garlic, minced
- 1 teaspoon ground cumin
- 1 teaspoon ground coriander
- 1 teaspoon ground cinnamon
- 1/2 teaspoon ground turmeric
- 1/2 teaspoon ground ginger
- 1/4 teaspoon cayenne pepper (optional, for added heat)
- Salt and pepper to taste
- 1/2 cup chicken broth (low sodium)
- 1/2 cup canned diced tomatoes
- 1/4 cup dried apricots, chopped
- 1/4 cup raisins or golden raisins
- 1/4 cup slivered almonds (optional, for garnish)
- 2 tablespoons fresh cilantro or parsley, chopped (optional, for garnish)

For the Couscous:

- 1 cup couscous (regular or whole wheat)
- 1 cup water or chicken broth (low sodium)
- 1 tablespoon olive oil
- Salt to taste

Instructions:

1. **Prepare the Chicken:**
   - o   In a large skillet or saucepan, heat the olive oil over medium heat. Add the chopped onion and sauté for 3-4 minutes until softened. Add the minced garlic and cook for an additional 1 minute until fragrant.
2. **Cook the Chicken:**
   - o   Add the chicken pieces to the skillet and season with cumin, coriander, cinnamon, turmeric, ground ginger, cayenne pepper (if using), salt, and pepper. Cook for 5-7 minutes, stirring occasionally, until the chicken is browned on all sides.
3. **Add the Liquid and Simmer:**
   - o   Stir in the chicken broth, diced tomatoes, chopped dried apricots, and raisins. Bring the mixture to a simmer, then reduce the heat to low and cover. Let it simmer for 15-20 minutes, or until the chicken is cooked through and the flavors have melded together.
4. **Prepare the Couscous:**
   - o   While the chicken is simmering, prepare the couscous. In a medium

saucepan, bring water or chicken broth
to a boil. Add a pinch of salt and 1
tablespoon of olive oil. Stir in the
couscous, cover, and remove from heat.
Let it sit for 5 minutes, then fluff with a
fork.

5. **Serve the Moroccan Chicken with Couscous:**
   o Divide the couscous among serving
     plates. Spoon the Moroccan chicken
     and sauce over the couscous.
6. **Garnish and Serve:**
   o Garnish with slivered almonds and
     fresh cilantro or parsley, if desired.

Snack: Pear Slices with Goat Cheese

Ingredients:

- 2 ripe pears, cored and sliced into wedges
- 1/4 cup goat cheese, crumbled
- 1 tablespoon honey or maple syrup (optional, for drizzling)
- 1 tablespoon walnuts or pecans, chopped (optional, for added crunch)
- A sprinkle of cinnamon (optional, for extra flavor)
- Fresh thyme or rosemary leaves (optional, for garnish)

Instructions:

1. **Prepare the Pear Slices:**
   o Wash and core the pears. Slice them
     into thin wedges or rounds, depending
     on your preference.
2. **Arrange the Pear Slices:**
   o Arrange the pear slices on a serving
     plate or platter.
3. **Add the Goat Cheese:**
   o Sprinkle the crumbled goat cheese
     evenly over the pear slices.
4. **Optional Toppings:**
   o Drizzle honey or maple syrup over the
     pear slices and goat cheese for a touch
     of sweetness, if desired.
   o Sprinkle chopped walnuts or pecans
     over the top for added crunch and
     texture.
   o Add a light sprinkle of cinnamon for
     extra flavor.
5. **Garnish (Optional):**
   o Garnish with fresh thyme or rosemary
     leaves for a pop of color and added
     aroma, if desired.

Dessert: Pumpkin Pie

Ingredients:

For the Crust:

- 1 1/4 cups all-purpose flour (or gluten-free flour blend)
- 1/2 teaspoon salt
- 1 tablespoon granulated sugar
- 1/2 cup cold unsalted butter, cut into small cubes
- 3-4 tablespoons ice water

For the Pumpkin Filling:

- 1 can (15 ounces) pumpkin puree
- 3/4 cup brown sugar
- 1 teaspoon ground cinnamon
- 1/2 teaspoon ground ginger
- 1/4 teaspoon ground nutmeg

- 1/4 teaspoon ground cloves
- 1/2 teaspoon salt
- 2 large eggs
- 1 cup heavy cream (or coconut milk for a dairy-free option)
- 1 teaspoon vanilla extract

Instructions:

1. **Prepare the Crust:**
   - In a large mixing bowl, whisk together the flour, salt, and granulated sugar. Add the cold, cubed butter and use a pastry cutter or your fingers to cut the butter into the flour mixture until it resembles coarse crumbs.
   - Gradually add the ice water, one tablespoon at a time, mixing until the dough starts to come together. Form the dough into a ball, wrap it in plastic wrap, and refrigerate for at least 30 minutes.
2. **Preheat the Oven:**
   - Preheat your oven to 375°F (190°C).
3. **Roll Out the Crust:**
   - On a lightly floured surface, roll out the chilled dough into a circle about 12 inches in diameter. Carefully transfer the dough to a 9-inch pie dish, pressing it gently into the bottom and sides. Trim any excess dough from the edges and crimp the edges with your fingers or a fork.
4. **Prepare the Pumpkin Filling:**
   - In a large mixing bowl, combine the pumpkin puree, brown sugar, cinnamon, ginger, nutmeg, cloves, and salt. Add the eggs and beat until smooth. Gradually add the heavy cream (or coconut milk) and vanilla extract, stirring until the filling is well mixed.
5. **Fill the Pie Crust:**
   - Pour the pumpkin filling into the prepared pie crust, spreading it out evenly with a spatula.
6. **Bake the Pie:**
   - Bake the pie in the preheated oven for 50-60 minutes, or until the filling is set and the crust is golden brown. To check for doneness, insert a knife or toothpick into the center of the pie; it should come out clean.
7. **Cool the Pie:**
   - Remove the pie from the oven and let it cool on a wire rack for at least 2 hours. This allows the filling to set completely.

Day 23

Breakfast: Cinnamon Raisin Overnight Oats

Ingredients:

- 1/2 cup rolled oats (use gluten-free oats if needed)
- 1/2 cup milk (dairy or dairy-free alternative, such as almond or oat milk)

- 1/4 cup Greek yogurt (or dairy-free yogurt alternative)
- 1 tablespoon chia seeds
- 1 tablespoon raisins
- 1/2 teaspoon ground cinnamon

- 1 tablespoon honey or maple syrup (optional, for added sweetness)

Optional Toppings:

- Fresh fruit (such as sliced bananas, berries, or apple slices)
- Chopped nuts (such as almonds, walnuts, or pecans)

- 1/4 teaspoon vanilla extract (optional)

- A drizzle of honey or maple syrup
- A sprinkle of additional ground cinnamon

Instructions:

1. **Combine the Ingredients:**
   o In a mason jar or a small bowl, combine the rolled oats, milk, Greek yogurt, chia seeds, raisins, ground cinnamon, honey or maple syrup (if using), and vanilla extract (if using).
2. **Mix Well:**
   o Stir the mixture well to ensure all the ingredients are evenly combined. Make sure the oats are fully submerged in the liquid.
3. **Refrigerate Overnight:**
   o Cover the jar or bowl with a lid or plastic wrap and refrigerate overnight (or for at least 4 hours). The oats will absorb the liquid and soften, creating a creamy, pudding-like consistency.
4. **Serve the Overnight Oats:**
   o In the morning, remove the oats from the refrigerator and give them a good stir. If the mixture is too thick, you can add a splash of milk to reach your desired consistency.
5. **Add Toppings (Optional):**
   o Top the overnight oats with fresh fruit, chopped nuts, a drizzle of honey or maple syrup, or an extra sprinkle of cinnamon, if desired.

Lunch: Grilled Chicken and Quinoa Bowl

Ingredients:

For the Grilled Chicken:

- 2 boneless, skinless chicken breasts
- 1 tablespoon olive oil
- 1 tablespoon lemon juice
- 1 teaspoon dried oregano
- 1/2 teaspoon garlic powder
- Salt and pepper to taste

For the Quinoa Bowl:

- 1 cup quinoa, rinsed
- 2 cups water or low-sodium chicken broth
- 1 cup cherry tomatoes, halved
- 1/2 cucumber, diced
- 1/2 red bell pepper, diced
- 1/4 red onion, thinly sliced

- 1/4 cup feta cheese, crumbled (optional)
- 1/4 cup fresh parsley or cilantro, chopped

For the Dressing:

- 3 tablespoons extra-virgin olive oil
- 2 tablespoons lemon juice
- 1 teaspoon Dijon mustard

- 2 tablespoons sliced almonds or sunflower seeds (optional, for added crunch)
- 1 teaspoon honey or maple syrup
- Salt and pepper to taste

Instructions:

1. **Marinate the Chicken:**
   - In a small bowl, combine the olive oil, lemon juice, dried oregano, garlic powder, salt, and pepper. Place the chicken breasts in a shallow dish or a resealable plastic bag and pour the marinade over them. Let the chicken marinate for at least 15 minutes, or up to 1 hour in the refrigerator.
2. **Cook the Quinoa:**
   - In a medium saucepan, bring the water or chicken broth to a boil. Add the rinsed quinoa, reduce the heat to low, cover, and simmer for about 15 minutes, or until the quinoa is tender and the liquid is absorbed. Remove from heat and let it sit, covered, for 5 minutes. Fluff with a fork and set aside to cool slightly.
3. **Grill the Chicken:**
   - Preheat a grill or grill pan over medium-high heat. Remove the chicken from the marinade and grill for about 5-7 minutes on each side, or until the chicken is cooked through and has reached an internal temperature of 165°F (75°C). Remove from the grill and let the chicken rest for a few minutes before slicing it into thin strips.
4. **Prepare the Dressing:**
   - In a small bowl, whisk together the extra-virgin olive oil, lemon juice, Dijon mustard, honey or maple syrup, salt, and pepper until well combined.
5. **Assemble the Quinoa Bowl:**
   - Divide the cooked quinoa among serving bowls. Top each bowl with the sliced grilled chicken, cherry tomatoes, cucumber, red bell pepper, red onion, feta cheese (if using), and fresh parsley or cilantro.
6. **Add the Dressing:**
   - Drizzle the dressing over each bowl and toss gently to combine.
7. **Add Toppings (Optional):**
   - Sprinkle with sliced almonds or sunflower seeds for added crunch, if desired.

Dinner: Lentil and Vegetable Curry

Ingredients:

For the Curry:

- 1 cup dried green or brown lentils, rinsed and drained
- 2 tablespoons olive oil
- 1 medium onion, finely chopped
- 3 cloves garlic, minced
- 1 tablespoon fresh ginger, grated
- 1 tablespoon curry powder
- 1 teaspoon ground cumin
- 1/2 teaspoon ground turmeric
- 1/2 teaspoon ground coriander

- 1/4 teaspoon cayenne pepper (optional, for heat)
- 1 medium carrot, diced
- 1 red bell pepper, diced
- 1 medium zucchini, diced
- 1 can (14 ounces) diced tomatoes
- 1 can (14 ounces) coconut milk (light or full fat)
- 2 cups vegetable broth or water
- Salt and pepper to taste
- 2 cups fresh spinach or kale, chopped

For Serving:

- Cooked brown or white rice, or quinoa
- Fresh cilantro, chopped (optional, for garnish)

- Lime wedges (optional, for serving)
- Plain Greek yogurt or dairy-free yogurt (optional, for serving)

Instructions:

1. **Cook the Lentils:**
   - In a medium saucepan, bring the vegetable broth or water to a boil. Add the lentils, reduce the heat to low, cover, and simmer for about 20-25 minutes, or until the lentils are tender but not mushy. Drain any excess liquid and set aside.
2. **Prepare the Curry Base:**
   - In a large pot or Dutch oven, heat the olive oil over medium heat. Add the chopped onion and sauté for 4-5 minutes, or until softened. Add the minced garlic and grated ginger and cook for another 1-2 minutes until fragrant.
3. **Add the Spices:**
   - Stir in the curry powder, cumin, turmeric, coriander, and cayenne pepper (if using). Cook for about 1 minute, stirring constantly, to toast the spices and enhance their flavors.
4. **Add the Vegetables:**
   - Add the diced carrot, red bell pepper, and zucchini to the pot. Stir to coat the vegetables in the spices, and cook for 3-4 minutes, or until they begin to soften.
5. **Add the Tomatoes and Coconut Milk:**
   - Pour in the diced tomatoes (with their juices) and coconut milk. Stir well to combine.
6. **Simmer the Curry:**
   - Add the cooked lentils to the pot, along with any remaining vegetable broth or water if needed to reach your desired consistency. Season with salt and pepper to taste. Bring the mixture to a simmer, cover, and cook for 15-20 minutes, or until the vegetables are tender and the flavors have melded together.
7. **Add the Greens:**
   - Stir in the chopped spinach or kale and cook for an additional 2-3 minutes, or until the greens are wilted.
8. **Serve the Curry:**
   - Serve the lentil and vegetable curry over a bed of cooked brown or white rice, or quinoa.
9. **Garnish and Serve:**
   - Garnish with fresh cilantro and serve with lime wedges and a dollop of Greek yogurt or dairy-free yogurt, if desired.

Snack: Roasted Beet Chips

Ingredients:

- 2-3 medium beets, peeled and thinly sliced (use a mandolin slicer for even slices)
- 1 tablespoon olive oil
- 1/2 teaspoon sea salt

- 1/4 teaspoon black pepper (optional, for added flavor)
- 1/4 teaspoon garlic powder (optional, for added flavor)
- 1/4 teaspoon smoked paprika (optional, for added flavor)

Instructions:

1. **Preheat the Oven:**
   - Preheat your oven to 350°F (175°C). Line two baking sheets with parchment paper or silicone baking mats.
2. **Prepare the Beets:**
   - Wash, peel, and thinly slice the beets into rounds, about 1/8-inch thick. Using a mandolin slicer will help ensure that all slices are the same thickness, which is important for even roasting.
3. **Season the Beets:**
   - In a large mixing bowl, toss the beet slices with olive oil until they are evenly coated. Sprinkle with sea salt, black pepper, garlic powder, and smoked paprika, if using. Toss again to coat the slices with the seasonings.
4. **Arrange on Baking Sheets:**
   - Arrange the beet slices in a single layer on the prepared baking sheets. Make sure the slices are not overlapping, as this will help them crisp up evenly.
5. **Roast the Beet Chips:**
   - Roast in the preheated oven for 20-30 minutes, or until the beet slices are crispy and slightly browned around the edges. Check them frequently, as the roasting time can vary depending on the thickness of the slices. Rotate the baking sheets halfway through the cooking time for even roasting.
6. **Cool the Beet Chips:**
   - Remove the baking sheets from the oven and let the beet chips cool on the baking sheets for a few minutes. They will continue to crisp up as they cool.

Dessert: Almond Butter Cookies

Ingredients:

- 1 cup almond butter (creamy or chunky, unsweetened)
- 1/2 cup granulated sugar or coconut sugar
- 1 large egg
- 1 teaspoon vanilla extract

- 1/2 teaspoon baking soda
- A pinch of salt
- 1/4 cup dark chocolate chips or chopped dark chocolate (optional)

Instructions:

1. **Preheat the Oven:**
   - Preheat your oven to 350°F (175°C). Line a baking sheet with parchment paper or a silicone baking mat.
2. **Prepare the Cookie Dough:**
   - In a large mixing bowl, combine the almond butter, granulated sugar, egg, vanilla extract, baking soda, and salt. Mix well until all ingredients are fully combined and a smooth dough forms. If

using chocolate chips or chopped dark
chocolate, fold them into the dough.

3. **Form the Cookies:**
   - Scoop tablespoon-sized portions of dough and roll them into balls. Place the dough balls onto the prepared baking sheet, spacing them about 2 inches apart. Use the back of a fork to gently press down on each ball, creating a crisscross pattern on top.
4. **Bake the Cookies:**
   - Bake the cookies in the preheated oven for 8-10 minutes, or until the edges are lightly golden. Be careful not to overbake, as the cookies will continue to firm up as they cool.
5. **Cool the Cookies:**
   - Remove the baking sheet from the oven and let the cookies cool on the sheet for 5 minutes before transferring them to a wire rack to cool completely.

Day 24

Breakfast: Chocolate Protein Smoothie

Ingredients:

- 1 ripe banana, frozen
- 1 cup unsweetened almond milk (or your preferred dairy-free milk)
- 1 scoop chocolate protein powder (whey, plant-based, or your choice)
- 1 tablespoon almond butter or peanut butter
- 1 tablespoon unsweetened cocoa powder
- 1 teaspoon honey or maple syrup (optional, for added sweetness)
- 1/2 teaspoon vanilla extract (optional)
- A handful of ice cubes (optional, for a thicker smoothie)

Optional Toppings:

- Sliced banana
- A sprinkle of cocoa nibs or dark chocolate shavings
- Chia seeds or flaxseeds (for added nutrition)

Instructions:

1. **Prepare the Ingredients:**
   - If you haven't already, freeze a ripe banana for a thicker, creamier texture in the smoothie.
2. **Blend the Smoothie:**
   - In a blender, combine the frozen banana, almond milk, chocolate protein powder, almond butter or peanut butter, cocoa powder, honey or maple syrup (if using), and vanilla extract (if using).
3. **Add Ice and Blend Until Smooth:**
   - Add a handful of ice cubes if you prefer a colder, thicker smoothie. Blend on high until all ingredients are fully combined and the smoothie is smooth and creamy.
4. **Serve the Smoothie:**
   - Pour the smoothie into a glass.
5. **Add Toppings (Optional):**
   - Top with sliced banana, a sprinkle of cocoa nibs or dark chocolate shavings, or chia seeds for added texture and nutrition

Lunch: Zoodle Salad with Lemon Tahini Dressing

Ingredients:

For the Salad:

- 2 medium zucchinis, spiralized into noodles (zoodles)
- 1 cup cherry tomatoes, halved
- 1/2 cucumber, thinly sliced
- 1/4 red onion, thinly sliced
- 1/2 red bell pepper, thinly sliced
- 1/4 cup Kalamata olives, pitted and halved
- 1/4 cup feta cheese, crumbled (optional)
- 2 tablespoons fresh parsley or cilantro, chopped (optional)

For the Lemon Tahini Dressing:

- 1/4 cup tahini (sesame seed paste)
- 3 tablespoons fresh lemon juice
- 1 tablespoon extra-virgin olive oil
- 1 tablespoon honey or maple syrup (optional, for added sweetness)
- 1 clove garlic, minced
- 2-3 tablespoons water (to thin the dressing to desired consistency)
- Salt and pepper to taste

Instructions:

1. **Prepare the Zoodles:**
   - Use a spiralizer to spiralize the zucchinis into noodles. If you don't have a spiralizer, you can use a julienne peeler or a regular vegetable peeler to create thin ribbons.
2. **Prepare the Salad Ingredients:**
   - In a large mixing bowl, combine the zoodles, halved cherry tomatoes, sliced cucumber, sliced red onion, sliced red bell pepper, Kalamata olives, and crumbled feta cheese (if using).
3. **Make the Lemon Tahini Dressing:**
   - In a small bowl, whisk together the tahini, fresh lemon juice, olive oil, honey or maple syrup (if using), minced garlic, salt, and pepper. Gradually add water, one tablespoon at a time, and whisk until the dressing reaches your desired consistency.
4. **Toss the Salad with Dressing:**
   - Drizzle the lemon tahini dressing over the salad ingredients in the bowl. Toss gently to combine, ensuring all the zoodles and vegetables are evenly coated with the dressing.
5. **Garnish and Serve:**
   - Garnish with fresh parsley or cilantro, if desired.

Dinner: Balsamic Glazed Pork Tenderloin

Ingredients:

For the Pork Tenderloin:

- 1 1/2 pounds pork tenderloin
- 1 tablespoon olive oil
- 1 teaspoon garlic powder
- 1 teaspoon dried rosemary
- 1/2 teaspoon salt
- 1/4 teaspoon black pepper

For the Balsamic Glaze:

- 1/2 cup balsamic vinegar
- 2 tablespoons honey or maple syrup
- 1 tablespoon Dijon mustard
- 1 clove garlic, minced
- Salt and pepper to taste

Instructions:

1. **Preheat the Oven:**
   - Preheat your oven to 400°F (200°C). Line a baking sheet with parchment paper or lightly grease it with olive oil.
2. **Season the Pork Tenderloin:**
   - In a small bowl, mix together the garlic powder, dried rosemary, salt, and black pepper. Rub the spice mixture all over the pork tenderloin.
3. **Sear the Pork Tenderloin:**
   - In a large skillet, heat the olive oil over medium-high heat. Add the pork tenderloin and sear on all sides until it is browned, about 2-3 minutes per side.
4. **Prepare the Balsamic Glaze:**
   - While the pork is searing, in a small saucepan, combine the balsamic vinegar, honey or maple syrup, Dijon mustard, and minced garlic. Bring to a simmer over medium heat and cook until the mixture has reduced by about half and thickened slightly, about 5-7 minutes. Season with salt and pepper to taste.
5. **Bake the Pork Tenderloin:**
   - Transfer the seared pork tenderloin to the prepared baking sheet. Brush generously with the balsamic glaze, reserving some for later. Place in the preheated oven and bake for 15-20 minutes, or until the internal temperature of the pork reaches 145°F (63°C).
6. **Rest and Slice the Pork:**
   - Remove the pork tenderloin from the oven and let it rest for 5-10 minutes before slicing. This allows the juices to redistribute and keeps the meat tender and juicy.

Snack: Fresh Pineapple Chunks

Ingredients:

- 1 fresh ripe pineapple

Optional Additions:

- A sprinkle of chili powder or Tajin seasoning (optional, for a spicy kick)

Instructions:

1. **Prepare the Pineapple:**
   - Place the pineapple on a cutting board. Using a sharp knife, cut off the top (crown) and the bottom of the pineapple.
   - Stand the pineapple upright and carefully slice off the outer skin, cutting downward in strips, following the curve of the fruit.
   - Remove any remaining "eyes" (the small, round, brown spots) with the tip of your knife.

2. **Cut the Pineapple into Chunks:**
   - Slice the pineapple in half lengthwise, then into quarters.

- A drizzle of honey or lime juice (optional, for added sweetness or tang)
- Fresh mint leaves (optional, for garnish)

   - Cut out the tough core from each quarter.
   - Slice each quarter into bite-sized chunks.

3. **Serve the Pineapple Chunks:**
   - Arrange the pineapple chunks on a serving plate or in a bowl.

4. **Add Optional Toppings:**
   - For added flavor, sprinkle a little chili powder or Tajin seasoning over the pineapple chunks for a spicy twist.
   - Drizzle with honey or a squeeze of fresh lime juice for a sweet and tangy flavor.
   - Garnish with fresh mint leaves for a refreshing touch.

Dessert: Mocha Mousse

Ingredients:

- 1/2 cup dark chocolate chips or chopped dark chocolate (70% cocoa or higher)
- 1 tablespoon instant espresso powder or instant coffee granules
- 2 tablespoons hot water

- 1 cup heavy whipping cream (or coconut cream for a dairy-free option)
- 2 tablespoons granulated sugar or honey (adjust to taste)
- 1 teaspoon vanilla extract
- A pinch of salt

Optional Toppings:

- Whipped cream or coconut whipped cream
- Chocolate shavings or cocoa nibs
- Fresh berries (such as raspberries or strawberries)

- A dusting of cocoa powder or powdered sugar
- Fresh mint leaves (for garnish)

Instructions:

1. **Melt the Chocolate:**

   - In a microwave-safe bowl or a heatproof bowl set over a pot of simmering water (double boiler), melt the dark chocolate chips or chopped

chocolate until smooth. Stir
occasionally to prevent burning. Once
melted, set aside to cool slightly.

2. **Dissolve the Espresso Powder:**
   o In a small bowl, dissolve the instant
     espresso powder or coffee granules in 2
     tablespoons of hot water. Stir until
     completely dissolved. Set aside to cool
     slightly.

3. **Whip the Cream:**
   o In a large mixing bowl, combine the
     heavy whipping cream, sugar or honey,
     vanilla extract, and a pinch of salt.
     Using an electric mixer, beat the cream
     on medium-high speed until soft peaks
     form.

4. **Add the Chocolate and Coffee Mixture:**
   o Gently fold the melted chocolate and
     dissolved coffee mixture into the
     whipped cream using a spatula. Be
     careful not to overmix; fold until just
     combined and the mixture is smooth
     and fluffy.

5. **Chill the Mousse:**
   o Spoon the mocha mousse into
     individual serving glasses or bowls.
     Cover and refrigerate for at least 1-2
     hours, or until the mousse is set and
     chilled.

6. **Serve the Mousse:**
   o Before serving, top each glass or bowl
     with whipped cream, chocolate
     shavings, fresh berries, or a dusting of
     cocoa powder, if desired. Garnish with
     fresh mint leaves for a pop of color.

Day 25

Breakfast: Berry Oatmeal Bake

Ingredients:

- 2 cups rolled oats (use gluten-free oats if needed)
- 1 teaspoon baking powder
- 1 teaspoon ground cinnamon
- 1/4 teaspoon salt
- 2 cups mixed berries (fresh or frozen, such as blueberries, strawberries, raspberries, and blackberries)
- 2 cups milk (dairy or dairy-free alternative, such as almond or oat milk)
- 1/4 cup maple syrup or honey
- 1 large egg
- 2 tablespoons melted coconut oil or unsalted butter
- 1 teaspoon vanilla extract
- 1/4 cup chopped nuts (such as almonds or walnuts, optional)
- 2 tablespoons chia seeds or flaxseeds (optional, for added fiber and nutrition)

Optional Toppings:

- Additional fresh berries
- A drizzle of maple syrup or honey
- Greek yogurt or dairy-free yogurt
- A sprinkle of chopped nuts

Instructions:

1. **Preheat the Oven:**
   o Preheat your oven to 375°F (190°C).
     Grease an 8x8-inch baking dish with
     coconut oil or butter.

2. **Prepare the Dry Ingredients:**
   o In a large mixing bowl, combine the
     rolled oats, baking powder, ground
     cinnamon, and salt. Stir to mix evenly.

3. **Add the Berries:**
   o Gently fold in the mixed berries and
     optional chia seeds or flaxseeds, if
     using, ensuring the berries are evenly
     distributed throughout the oat mixture.

4. **Mix the Wet Ingredients:**
   o In a separate bowl, whisk together the
     milk, maple syrup or honey, egg,

melted coconut oil or butter, and vanilla extract until well combined.

5. **Combine the Mixtures:**
   - Pour the wet ingredients over the dry oat and berry mixture. Stir gently to combine, making sure all the oats are moistened.
6. **Pour into the Baking Dish:**
   - Pour the oatmeal mixture into the prepared baking dish, spreading it out evenly.
7. **Add Toppings:**
   - Sprinkle the top with chopped nuts, if desired, for added crunch.
8. **Bake the Oatmeal:**
   - Bake in the preheated oven for 35-40 minutes, or until the oatmeal is set and the top is golden brown.
9. **Cool Slightly and Serve:**
   - Remove from the oven and let the oatmeal bake cool for a few minutes before serving.
10. **Add Optional Toppings:**
    - Serve warm with additional fresh berries, a drizzle of maple syrup or honey, a dollop of Greek yogurt or dairy-free yogurt, and a sprinkle of chopped nuts, if desired.

Lunch: Spicy Tuna Salad Wrap

Ingredients:

For the Spicy Tuna Salad:

- 1 can (5 ounces) tuna, drained (packed in water or olive oil)
- 2 tablespoons Greek yogurt (or mayonnaise for a richer flavor)
- 1 tablespoon Sriracha or your preferred hot sauce (adjust to taste)
- 1 teaspoon Dijon mustard
- 1/4 cup celery, finely chopped
- 1/4 cup red onion, finely chopped
- 1 tablespoon fresh parsley or cilantro, chopped (optional)
- Salt and pepper to taste
- 1/2 avocado, sliced (optional, for added creaminess)

For the Wrap:

- 2 large whole wheat or gluten-free tortillas
- 1 cup mixed greens or lettuce
- 1/2 cucumber, thinly sliced
- 1/2 carrot, shredded
- 1/4 cup shredded red cabbage (optional, for added crunch)
- 1/4 cup alfalfa sprouts (optional)

Instructions:

1. **Prepare the Spicy Tuna Salad:**
   - In a medium mixing bowl, combine the drained tuna, Greek yogurt (or mayonnaise), Sriracha or hot sauce, Dijon mustard, chopped celery, chopped red onion, and fresh parsley or cilantro (if using). Mix well until all ingredients are evenly combined. Season with salt and pepper to taste.
2. **Assemble the Wrap:**
   - Lay the tortillas flat on a clean surface. Place a handful of mixed greens or lettuce in the center of each tortilla.
3. **Add the Vegetables:**
   - Top the greens with sliced cucumber, shredded carrot, shredded red cabbage (if using), and alfalfa sprouts (if using).
4. **Add the Spicy Tuna Salad:**
   - Spoon the spicy tuna salad mixture over the vegetables in the center of each tortilla. If using, add slices of avocado on top of the tuna salad for added creaminess.

5. **Roll the Wraps:**

- o   Fold in the sides of each tortilla, then roll it up tightly from the bottom to enclose the filling.

Dinner: Grilled Steak with Roasted Vegetables

Ingredients:

For the Grilled Steak:

- 2 ribeye or sirloin steaks (about 6-8 ounces each)
- 1 tablespoon olive oil
- 2 cloves garlic, minced
- 1 teaspoon dried rosemary or thyme
- Salt and pepper to taste

For the Roasted Vegetables:

- 1 red bell pepper, sliced
- 1 yellow bell pepper, sliced
- 1 zucchini, sliced into rounds
- 1 red onion, cut into wedges
- 1 cup cherry tomatoes
- 1 tablespoon olive oil
- 1 teaspoon dried Italian seasoning (or a mix of dried basil, oregano, and thyme)
- Salt and pepper to taste

Instructions:

1. **Preheat the Oven for Roasted Vegetables:**
    - o   Preheat your oven to 400°F (200°C). Line a large baking sheet with parchment paper or a silicone baking mat.
2. **Prepare the Roasted Vegetables:**
    - o   In a large mixing bowl, combine the sliced bell peppers, zucchini, red onion wedges, and cherry tomatoes. Drizzle with olive oil and sprinkle with Italian seasoning, salt, and pepper. Toss to coat the vegetables evenly.
3. **Roast the Vegetables:**
    - o   Spread the vegetables in a single layer on the prepared baking sheet. Roast in the preheated oven for 20-25 minutes, or until the vegetables are tender and slightly caramelized, stirring halfway through to ensure even cooking.
4. **Prepare the Steaks:**
    - o   While the vegetables are roasting, prepare the steaks. In a small bowl, mix the olive oil, minced garlic, dried rosemary or thyme, salt, and pepper. Rub the mixture evenly over both sides of the steaks.
5. **Grill the Steaks:**
    - o   Preheat a grill or grill pan over medium-high heat. Once hot, place the steaks on the grill and cook for 4-6 minutes per side for medium-rare, or adjust the cooking time according to your preferred level of doneness. Use a meat thermometer to check the internal temperature: 130°F (54°C) for medium-rare, 140°F (60°C) for medium, or 150°F (66°C) for well done.

6. **Rest the Steaks:**
   - o Remove the steaks from the grill and let them rest on a cutting board, loosely covered with foil, for about 5-10 minutes to allow the juices to redistribute.
7. **Serve the Dish:**
   - o Slice the steaks against the grain into thin strips. Arrange the grilled steak slices and roasted vegetables on serving plates.
8. **Optional Garnish:**
   - o Garnish with fresh herbs, such as parsley or rosemary, if desired.

Snack: Sunflower Seeds

Ingredients:

- 1/2 cup sunflower seeds (shelled, unsalted)
- Optional seasonings:
  - o A pinch of sea salt
  - o A dash of paprika or cayenne pepper (for a spicy kick)
  - o A sprinkle of garlic powder or onion powder (for added flavor)

Instructions:

1. **Prepare the Sunflower Seeds:**
   - o If you prefer flavored sunflower seeds, mix the seeds with your choice of seasonings in a small bowl. Toss to coat the seeds evenly.
2. **Toast the Sunflower Seeds (Optional):**
   - o To enhance the flavor, you can toast the sunflower seeds. Preheat a dry skillet over medium heat. Add the sunflower seeds and toast them for 3-5 minutes, stirring frequently to prevent burning. Toast until they are golden brown and fragrant.
3. **Cool the Seeds:**
   - o Remove the skillet from the heat and let the toasted sunflower seeds cool completely.
4. **Serve the Sunflower Seeds:**
   - o Once cooled, serve the sunflower seeds in a small bowl.

Dessert: Pomegranate Sorbet

Ingredients:

- 2 cups pomegranate juice (fresh or store-bought, 100% juice)
- 1/2 cup water
- 1/2 cup granulated sugar or honey (adjust to taste)
- 1 tablespoon fresh lemon juice
- Pomegranate seeds (arils) for garnish (optional)
- Fresh mint leaves for garnish (optional)

Instructions:

1. **Prepare the Simple Syrup:**
   - In a small saucepan, combine the water and sugar (or honey). Heat over medium heat, stirring constantly, until the sugar is completely dissolved. Once dissolved, remove from heat and let the simple syrup cool to room temperature.
2. **Combine the Ingredients:**
   - In a mixing bowl, combine the pomegranate juice, cooled simple syrup, and fresh lemon juice. Stir well to combine.
3. **Chill the Mixture:**
   - Cover the bowl with plastic wrap and refrigerate the mixture for at least 1-2 hours, or until thoroughly chilled.
4. **Churn the Sorbet:**
   - Pour the chilled pomegranate mixture into an ice cream maker and churn according to the manufacturer's instructions, usually about 20-25 minutes, or until the sorbet reaches a soft, scoopable consistency.
5. **Freeze the Sorbet:**
   - Transfer the churned sorbet to an airtight container and freeze for at least 2-4 hours, or until firm.
6. **Serve the Sorbet:**
   - Scoop the pomegranate sorbet into bowls or cups.
7. **Garnish and Enjoy:**
   - Garnish with fresh pomegranate seeds and mint leaves if desired. Serve immediately.

Day 26

Breakfast: Avocado and Veggie Toast

Ingredients:

- 2 slices whole grain or gluten-free bread
- 1 ripe avocado
- 1/2 teaspoon fresh lemon juice
- Salt and pepper to taste
- 1/4 cup cherry tomatoes, halved
- 1/4 cucumber, thinly sliced
- 1/4 red bell pepper, thinly sliced
- 1/4 cup sprouts or microgreens (optional)
- 1 tablespoon feta cheese, crumbled (optional)
- A sprinkle of red pepper flakes (optional, for added heat)
- Fresh herbs (such as cilantro, parsley, or basil) for garnish (optional)

Instructions:

1. **Toast the Bread:**
   - Toast the slices of whole grain or gluten-free bread in a toaster or under a broiler until golden and crispy.
2. **Prepare the Avocado Spread:**
   - While the bread is toasting, cut the avocado in half, remove the pit, and scoop the flesh into a small bowl. Add the fresh lemon juice, salt, and pepper. Mash the avocado with a fork until smooth and creamy.
3. **Spread the Avocado:**
   - Spread the mashed avocado evenly over each slice of toasted bread.
4. **Add the Veggies:**
   - Top the avocado spread with halved cherry tomatoes, thinly sliced cucumber, and red bell pepper.
5. **Add Optional Toppings:**
   - Sprinkle with sprouts or microgreens, feta cheese (if using), and red pepper flakes for added flavor and texture. Garnish with fresh herbs like cilantro, parsley, or basil for extra freshness, if desired.

Lunch: Cauliflower Rice and Veggie Stir-Fry

Ingredients:

For the Cauliflower Rice:

- 1 medium head of cauliflower, cut into florets
- 1 tablespoon olive oil
- Salt and pepper to taste

For the Veggie Stir-Fry:

- 1 tablespoon olive oil or sesame oil
- 1/2 red bell pepper, thinly sliced
- 1/2 yellow bell pepper, thinly sliced
- 1 cup snap peas or green beans, trimmed
- 1 medium carrot, julienned or thinly sliced
- 1/2 cup mushrooms, sliced
- 2 cloves garlic, minced
- 1 tablespoon fresh ginger, grated
- 2 tablespoons low-sodium soy sauce or tamari (for gluten-free option)
- 1 tablespoon rice vinegar
- 1 tablespoon sesame seeds (optional, for garnish)
- 2 tablespoons green onions, sliced (optional, for garnish)
- Fresh cilantro or parsley, chopped (optional, for garnish)

Instructions:

1. **Prepare the Cauliflower Rice:**
   - Place the cauliflower florets in a food processor and pulse until they reach a rice-like consistency. Be careful not to over-process, or you may end up with cauliflower mush.
2. **Cook the Cauliflower Rice:**
   - In a large skillet, heat 1 tablespoon of olive oil over medium heat. Add the cauliflower rice, season with salt and pepper, and sauté for 5-7 minutes, or until the cauliflower is tender but not mushy. Remove from heat and set aside.
3. **Prepare the Veggie Stir-Fry:**
   - In the same skillet or a wok, heat 1 tablespoon of olive oil or sesame oil over medium-high heat. Add the sliced bell peppers, snap peas or green beans, julienned carrot, and mushrooms. Stir-fry for 4-5 minutes, or until the vegetables are tender-crisp.
4. **Add Garlic and Ginger:**
   - Add the minced garlic and grated ginger to the skillet and stir-fry for another 1-2 minutes until fragrant.
5. **Add the Sauce:**
   - Stir in the low-sodium soy sauce or tamari and rice vinegar. Cook for an additional 2-3 minutes, allowing the flavors to combine.
6. **Combine the Stir-Fry with Cauliflower Rice:**
   - Add the cooked cauliflower rice to the skillet with the vegetables. Stir to combine and heat through for 1-2 minutes.
7. **Garnish and Serve:**
   - Garnish the stir-fry with sesame seeds, sliced green onions, and fresh cilantro or parsley, if desired.

Dinner: Herb-Crusted Salmon with Quinoa Pilaf

Ingredients:

For the Herb-Crusted Salmon:

- 4 salmon fillets (about 6 ounces each)
- 2 tablespoons olive oil
- 1/2 cup panko breadcrumbs (or gluten-free breadcrumbs)
- 1/4 cup fresh parsley, finely chopped
- 1 tablespoon fresh dill, finely chopped
- 1 tablespoon fresh thyme, finely chopped
- 2 cloves garlic, minced
- Zest of 1 lemon
- Salt and pepper to taste

For the Quinoa Pilaf:

- 1 cup quinoa, rinsed
- 2 cups low-sodium vegetable or chicken broth
- 1 tablespoon olive oil
- 1/2 onion, finely chopped
- 1 clove garlic, minced
- 1/2 cup carrots, finely diced
- 1/2 cup celery, finely diced
- 1/4 cup slivered almonds or chopped nuts (optional)
- 1/4 cup dried cranberries or raisins (optional)
- 1/4 cup fresh parsley, chopped
- Salt and pepper to taste

Instructions:

1. **Preheat the Oven:**
   - Preheat your oven to 400°F (200°C). Line a baking sheet with parchment paper or lightly grease it with olive oil.
2. **Prepare the Herb-Crusted Salmon:**
   - In a small bowl, mix the panko breadcrumbs, chopped parsley, dill, thyme, minced garlic, lemon zest, salt, and pepper. Add 2 tablespoons of olive oil and mix until the breadcrumb mixture is well coated.
   - Place the salmon fillets on the prepared baking sheet. Press the breadcrumb mixture evenly on top of each salmon fillet, pressing gently to adhere.
3. **Bake the Salmon:**
   - Bake in the preheated oven for 12-15 minutes, or until the salmon is cooked through and the crust is golden and crispy. The internal temperature should reach 145°F (63°C).
4. **Prepare the Quinoa Pilaf:**
   - While the salmon is baking, prepare the quinoa pilaf. In a medium saucepan, heat 1 tablespoon of olive oil over medium heat. Add the chopped onion, garlic, carrots, and celery. Sauté for 3-4 minutes, or until the vegetables are softened.
5. **Cook the Quinoa:**
   - Add the rinsed quinoa to the saucepan and stir to coat with the vegetable mixture. Pour in the vegetable or chicken broth, bring to a boil, then reduce the heat to low. Cover and simmer for about 15 minutes, or until the quinoa is tender and the liquid is absorbed.
6. **Finish the Quinoa Pilaf:**
   - Remove the quinoa from heat and fluff with a fork. Stir in the slivered almonds or chopped nuts and dried cranberries or raisins, if using. Season with salt and pepper to taste. Garnish with fresh parsley.
7. **Serve the Dish:**
   - Divide the quinoa pilaf among serving plates. Place the herb-crusted salmon fillets on top or beside the quinoa pilaf.

Snack: Orange Slices with Dark Chocolate

Ingredients:

- 2 medium oranges, peeled and segmented
- 1/2 cup dark chocolate (70% cocoa or higher), chopped or use dark chocolate chips
- 1/2 teaspoon sea salt (optional, for garnish)

Instructions:

1. **Prepare the Orange Slices:**
   - Peel the oranges and separate them into individual segments. Remove any remaining pith from the segments for a clean presentation.
2. **Melt the Dark Chocolate:**
   - In a microwave-safe bowl or using a double boiler, melt the dark chocolate until smooth. If using a microwave, heat in 30-second intervals, stirring between each interval to prevent burning.
3. **Dip the Orange Slices:**
   - Dip each orange segment halfway into the melted dark chocolate, letting any excess chocolate drip off. Place the dipped orange slices on a parchment-lined baking sheet.
4. **Add Optional Garnish:**
   - Sprinkle a small pinch of sea salt over the chocolate-dipped part of each orange slice for a contrasting flavor, if desired.
5. **Chill the Orange Slices:**
   - Place the baking sheet in the refrigerator for about 15-20 minutes, or until the chocolate is set.

Dessert: Honeydew Melon Sorbet

Ingredients:

- 4 cups honeydew melon, cubed (about 1 medium honeydew melon)
- 1/4 cup honey or maple syrup (adjust to taste)
- 2 tablespoons fresh lime juice
- 1/4 cup water
- Fresh mint leaves (optional, for garnish)

Instructions:

1. **Prepare the Honeydew Melon:**
   - Cut the honeydew melon in half and remove the seeds. Scoop out the flesh and cut it into cubes. Measure out 4 cups of cubed melon and place them in a single layer on a baking sheet. Freeze the melon cubes for at least 2-3 hours, or until fully frozen.
2. **Blend the Sorbet Mixture:**
   - In a blender or food processor, combine the frozen honeydew melon cubes, honey or maple syrup, fresh lime juice, and water. Blend until smooth and creamy, stopping to scrape down the sides as needed.
3. **Adjust Sweetness:**
   - Taste the sorbet mixture and adjust the sweetness by adding more honey or maple syrup, if desired. Blend again to incorporate.
4. **Chill the Sorbet:**

- o Transfer the blended mixture to a loaf pan or airtight container. Smooth the top with a spatula and cover with plastic wrap or a lid. Freeze for at least 1-2 hours, or until the sorbet is firm enough to scoop.

5. **Serve the Sorbet:**
   - o Scoop the honeydew melon sorbet into bowls or cups using an ice cream scoop.
6. **Garnish and Enjoy:**
   - o Garnish with fresh mint leaves, if desired, for added color and a refreshing touch.

Day 27

Breakfast: Spinach and Feta Frittata

Ingredients:

- 8 large eggs
- 1/4 cup milk (dairy or dairy-free alternative)
- 1 tablespoon olive oil
- 1/2 cup onion, finely chopped
- 2 cloves garlic, minced
- 2 cups fresh spinach, chopped
- 1/2 cup cherry tomatoes, halved
- 1/2 cup feta cheese, crumbled
- Salt and pepper to taste
- Fresh herbs (such as parsley or dill) for garnish (optional)

Instructions:

1. **Preheat the Oven:**
   - o Preheat your oven to 375°F (190°C).
2. **Prepare the Egg Mixture:**
   - o In a large mixing bowl, whisk together the eggs, milk, salt, and pepper until well combined. Set aside.
3. **Sauté the Vegetables:**
   - o Heat the olive oil in an ovenproof skillet or cast-iron pan over medium heat. Add the chopped onion and sauté for 3-4 minutes, or until softened. Add the minced garlic and cook for an additional 1 minute, until fragrant.
4. **Add Spinach and Tomatoes:**
   - o Add the chopped spinach to the skillet and sauté for 2-3 minutes, or until wilted. Add the halved cherry tomatoes and cook for another 1-2 minutes.
5. **Combine the Ingredients:**
   - o Pour the egg mixture over the sautéed vegetables in the skillet, ensuring that the vegetables are evenly distributed. Sprinkle the crumbled feta cheese over the top.
6. **Cook the Frittata:**
   - o Cook on the stovetop over medium heat for about 2-3 minutes, or until the edges of the frittata begin to set.
7. **Bake the Frittata:**
   - o Transfer the skillet to the preheated oven and bake for 10-12 minutes, or until the frittata is fully set and lightly golden on top. The center should be firm and not jiggly.
8. **Cool and Serve:**
   - o Remove the frittata from the oven and let it cool for a few minutes before slicing.
9. **Garnish and Serve:**
   - o Garnish with fresh herbs, if desired, and serve warm.

Lunch: Grilled Vegetable and Hummus Wrap

Ingredients:

- 1 large whole wheat or gluten-free tortilla
- 1/2 cup hummus (store-bought or homemade)
- 1/2 red bell pepper, thinly sliced
- 1/2 zucchini, sliced into thin rounds
- 1/2 yellow squash, sliced into thin rounds
- 1/4 red onion, thinly sliced
- 1/4 cup baby spinach leaves

- 1/4 cup feta cheese, crumbled (optional)
- 1 tablespoon olive oil
- Salt and pepper to taste
- 1 teaspoon balsamic vinegar (optional, for drizzling)
- Fresh herbs (such as basil or parsley) for garnish (optional)

Instructions:

1. **Preheat the Grill:**
   - Preheat a grill or grill pan over medium-high heat.
2. **Prepare the Vegetables:**
   - In a bowl, toss the sliced bell pepper, zucchini, yellow squash, and red onion with olive oil, salt, and pepper until evenly coated.
3. **Grill the Vegetables:**
   - Place the vegetables on the preheated grill or grill pan. Cook for 2-3 minutes per side, or until the vegetables are tender and have nice grill marks. Remove from the grill and set aside.
4. **Assemble the Wrap:**
   - Lay the tortilla flat on a clean surface. Spread a generous layer of hummus over the entire surface of the tortilla.
5. **Add the Grilled Vegetables:**
   - Arrange the grilled vegetables evenly over the hummus.
6. **Add the Spinach and Feta:**
   - Top with baby spinach leaves and sprinkle with crumbled feta cheese (if using).
7. **Drizzle with Balsamic Vinegar (Optional):**
   - Drizzle with balsamic vinegar for extra flavor, if desired.
8. **Roll the Wrap:**
   - Fold in the sides of the tortilla and then roll it up tightly from the bottom to enclose the filling.

Dinner: Chicken and Vegetable Kebabs

Ingredients:

For the Chicken and Vegetable Kebabs:

- 1-pound boneless, skinless chicken breast, cut into 1-inch cubes
- 1 red bell pepper, cut into 1-inch pieces
- 1 yellow bell pepper, cut into 1-inch pieces
- 1 red onion, cut into 1-inch pieces
- 1 zucchini, sliced into 1/2-inch rounds
- 1 cup cherry tomatoes
- 2 tablespoons olive oil

- 2 tablespoons lemon juice
- 2 cloves garlic, minced
- 1 teaspoon dried oregano
- 1/2 teaspoon paprika
- Salt and pepper to taste
- Wooden or metal skewers (if using wooden skewers, soak them in water for at least 30 minutes to prevent burning)

Optional Garnish:

- Fresh parsley or cilantro, chopped

- Lemon wedges

Instructions:

1. **Prepare the Marinade:**
   o In a large bowl, combine the olive oil, lemon juice, minced garlic, dried oregano, paprika, salt, and pepper. Mix well to create a marinade.
2. **Marinate the Chicken:**
   o Add the cubed chicken pieces to the marinade and toss to coat evenly. Cover and refrigerate for at least 30 minutes to 1 hour to allow the flavors to meld.
3. **Prepare the Vegetables:**
   o While the chicken is marinating, prepare the vegetables by cutting them into 1-inch pieces. Keep the cherry tomatoes whole.
4. **Assemble the Kebabs:**
   o Preheat your grill or grill pan over medium-high heat. Thread the marinated chicken and vegetables onto skewers, alternating between the chicken, bell peppers, onion, zucchini, and cherry tomatoes.
5. **Grill the Kebabs:**
   o Place the kebabs on the preheated grill and cook for 10-15 minutes, turning occasionally, until the chicken is cooked through, and the vegetables are tender and slightly charred. The chicken should reach an internal temperature of 165°F (74°C).
6. **Serve the Kebabs:**
   o Remove the kebabs from the grill and transfer them to a serving platter.
7. **Garnish and Serve:**
   o Garnish with fresh parsley or cilantro and serve with lemon wedges for squeezing over the kebabs.

Snack: Popcorn with Nutritional Yeast

Ingredients:

- 1/4 cup popcorn kernels
- 1 tablespoon olive oil or coconut oil
- 2 tablespoons nutritional yeast
- 1/4 teaspoon sea salt (adjust to taste)
- 1/4 teaspoon garlic powder (optional, for added flavor)
- 1/4 teaspoon paprika or cayenne pepper (optional, for a spicy kick)

Instructions:

1. **Heat the Oil:**
   o In a large, heavy-bottomed pot with a lid, heat the olive oil or coconut oil over medium heat. Add a few popcorn kernels to the pot and cover with the lid. When the test kernels pop, the oil is hot enough.
2. **Pop the Popcorn:**
   o Add the rest of the popcorn kernels to the pot and cover with the lid. Shake the pot gently to coat the kernels with oil. Continue to shake the pot occasionally as the kernels begin to pop. Keep the lid slightly ajar to allow steam to escape.
3. **Finish Popping:**
   o Once the popping slows to about 2-3 seconds between pops, remove the pot from the heat. Keep the lid on for a few moments to allow any last kernels to pop.
4. **Season the Popcorn:**
   o Immediately transfer the popcorn to a large mixing bowl. Sprinkle the nutritional yeast, sea salt, garlic powder (if using), and paprika or cayenne pepper (if using) over the popcorn. Toss well to evenly distribute the seasonings.

Dessert: Apricot Tart

Ingredients:

For the Crust:

- 1 1/4 cups all-purpose flour (or gluten-free flour blend)
- 1/4 cup granulated sugar
- 1/4 teaspoon salt
- 1/2 cup cold unsalted butter, cut into small cubes
- 2-3 tablespoons ice water

For the Filling:

- 6-8 fresh apricots, halved and pitted
- 1/4 cup granulated sugar
- 1 tablespoon cornstarch
- 1 tablespoon fresh lemon juice
- 1 teaspoon vanilla extract
- 1/4 cup apricot jam or preserves (optional, for glaze)

For the Topping:

- 2 tablespoons sliced almonds (optional)
- 1 tablespoon powdered sugar (optional, for dusting)

Instructions:

1. **Prepare the Crust:**
   - In a large mixing bowl, combine the flour, granulated sugar, and salt. Add the cold butter cubes and use a pastry cutter or your fingers to cut the butter into the flour mixture until it resembles coarse crumbs.
2. **Form the Dough:**
   - Gradually add ice water, one tablespoon at a time, mixing until the dough comes together. Form the dough into a ball, flatten it into a disk, wrap it in plastic wrap, and refrigerate for at least 30 minutes.
3. **Preheat the Oven:**
   - Preheat your oven to 375°F (190°C). Line a baking sheet with parchment paper.
4. **Roll Out the Dough:**
   - On a lightly floured surface, roll out the chilled dough into a circle about 12 inches in diameter. Carefully transfer the dough to a tart pan or lay it flat on the prepared baking sheet for a more rustic, free-form tart.
5. **Prepare the Apricot Filling:**
   - In a large bowl, combine the halved apricots, granulated sugar, cornstarch, lemon juice, and vanilla extract. Toss gently to coat the apricots evenly.
6. **Assemble the Tart:**
   - Arrange the apricot halves, cut side up, in a circular pattern over the rolled-out dough, leaving a 1–2-inch border around the edges. Fold the edges of the dough over the apricots to create a rustic edge.
7. **Add Optional Toppings:**
   - Sprinkle the tart with sliced almonds, if using, for added crunch.
8. **Bake the Tart:**
   - Bake in the preheated oven for 30-35 minutes, or until the crust is golden brown and the apricots are tender and bubbling.
9. **Glaze the Tart (Optional):**
   - If desired, warm the apricot jam or preserves in a small saucepan over low heat until it becomes liquid. Brush the warm jam over the apricots to create a glossy finish.

10. **Cool and Serve:**
    o   Allow the tart to cool for a few minutes before transferring it to a wire rack. Dust with powdered sugar before serving, if desired.

Day 28

Breakfast: Apple Cinnamon Muffins

Ingredients:

- 1 1/2 cups all-purpose flour (or whole wheat flour for a healthier option)
- 1/2 cup rolled oats
- 1/2 cup granulated sugar or coconut sugar
- 1 teaspoon baking powder
- 1/2 teaspoon baking soda
- 1/2 teaspoon salt
- 1 teaspoon ground cinnamon
- 1/4 teaspoon ground nutmeg
- 2 large eggs
- 1/2 cup unsweetened applesauce
- 1/4 cup coconut oil or vegetable oil, melted
- 1/2 cup milk (dairy or dairy-free alternative, such as almond or oat milk)
- 1 teaspoon vanilla extract
- 1 1/2 cups apple, peeled and diced (about 1 large apple)
- 1/4 cup chopped walnuts or pecans (optional)

Instructions:

1. **Preheat the Oven:**
   o   Preheat your oven to 375°F (190°C). Line a 12-cup muffin tin with paper liners or lightly grease it with cooking spray.
2. **Prepare the Dry Ingredients:**
   o   In a large mixing bowl, combine the flour, rolled oats, sugar, baking powder, baking soda, salt, ground cinnamon, and ground nutmeg. Whisk together until well combined.
3. **Mix the Wet Ingredients:**
   o   In a separate bowl, whisk together the eggs, applesauce, melted coconut oil, milk, and vanilla extract until smooth.
4. **Combine the Mixtures:**
   o   Pour the wet ingredients into the dry ingredients and stir gently until just combined. Do not overmix; a few lumps are okay. Fold in the diced apples and chopped nuts (if using).
5. **Fill the Muffin Cups:**
   o   Divide the batter evenly among the muffin cups, filling each about 2/3 full.
6. **Bake the Muffins:**
   o   Bake in the preheated oven for 18-22 minutes, or until a toothpick inserted into the center of a muffin comes out clean.
7. **Cool the Muffins:**
   o   Remove the muffins from the oven and let them cool in the pan for 5 minutes. Then transfer them to a wire rack to cool completely.

Lunch: Kale Caesar Salad with Grilled Chicken

Ingredients:

For the Salad:

- 2 large chicken breasts, grilled and sliced
- 4 cups kale, tough stems removed, and leaves chopped
- 2 cups romaine lettuce, chopped

- 1/4 cup Parmesan cheese, grated or shaved
- 1/2 cup croutons (optional)
- 1/4 cup cherry tomatoes, halved (optional)

For the Caesar Dressing:

- 1/4 cup plain Greek yogurt
- 2 tablespoons olive oil
- 1 tablespoon lemon juice
- 1 teaspoon Dijon mustard
- 1 teaspoon Worcestershire sauce

- 1 small garlic clove, minced
- 1/4 cup grated Parmesan cheese
- Salt and pepper to taste

Instructions:

1. **Prepare the Dressing:**
   - In a small bowl, whisk together the Greek yogurt, olive oil, lemon juice, Dijon mustard, Worcestershire sauce, minced garlic, grated Parmesan cheese, salt, and pepper until smooth and well combined. Set aside.

2. **Massage the Kale:**
   - In a large mixing bowl, add the chopped kale and a small drizzle of olive oil or a splash of the dressing. Use your hands to gently massage the kale for about 2-3 minutes until the leaves become softer and darker. This process makes the kale more tender and easier to eat.

3. **Assemble the Salad:**
   - Add the chopped romaine lettuce to the bowl with the massaged kale. Toss to combine. Add the grilled chicken slices, grated or shaved Parmesan cheese, and croutons (if using). If desired, add halved cherry tomatoes for extra color and flavor.

4. **Dress the Salad:**
   - Drizzle the Caesar dressing over the salad and toss gently to coat all the ingredients evenly. Start with half the dressing and add more as needed to suit your taste.

5. **Serve the Salad:**
   - Divide the kale Caesar salad with grilled chicken among serving plates.

6. **Garnish and Enjoy:**
   - Garnish with extra Parmesan cheese, freshly ground black pepper, or additional croutons, if desired.

Dinner: Seared Tuna with Mango Salsa

Ingredients:

For the Seared Tuna:

- 4 tuna steaks (about 6 ounces each)
- 2 tablespoons olive oil
- Salt and pepper to taste

- 1 teaspoon sesame seeds (optional, for garnish)
- 1 lime, cut into wedges (for serving)

For the Mango Salsa:

- 1 ripe mango, peeled, pitted, and diced
- 1/2 red bell pepper, diced
- 1/4 red onion, finely chopped
- 1/2 jalapeño, seeded and finely chopped (optional, for heat)
- 2 tablespoons fresh cilantro, chopped

- 1 tablespoon fresh lime juice
- 1/4 teaspoon salt
- 1/4 teaspoon black pepper

Instructions:

1. **Prepare the Mango Salsa:**
   - In a medium bowl, combine the diced mango, red bell pepper, red onion, jalapeño (if using), fresh cilantro, lime juice, salt, and pepper. Toss gently to mix all the ingredients. Cover and refrigerate the salsa while you prepare the tuna to allow the flavors to meld.
2. **Season the Tuna Steaks:**
   - Pat the tuna steaks dry with a paper towel. Drizzle with olive oil and season both sides with salt and pepper.
3. **Sear the Tuna Steaks:**
   - Heat a large skillet or grill pan over medium-high heat. Once the pan is hot, add the tuna steaks. Sear for about 1-2 minutes per side for rare to medium-rare, depending on your preference. The outside should be nicely browned while the inside remains pink. Adjust cooking time if you prefer your tuna more well-done.
4. **Serve the Tuna:**
   - Transfer the seared tuna steaks to serving plates.
5. **Top with Mango Salsa:**
   - Spoon the chilled mango salsa over each tuna steak.
6. **Garnish and Serve:**
   - Garnish with sesame seeds (if using) and serve with lime wedges on the side for squeezing over the tuna.

Snack: Dried Apricots and Almonds

Ingredients:

- 1/2 cup dried apricots

- 1/4 cup whole almonds (raw or lightly roasted, unsalted)

Instructions:

1. **Prepare the Snack:**
   - Measure out the dried apricots and almonds.
2. **Serve the Snack:**
   - Arrange the dried apricots and almonds on a small serving plate or in a bowl.

Dessert: Tiramisu

Ingredients:

For the Cream Layer:

- 1 cup heavy cream, cold
- 1 cup mascarpone cheese, softened
- 1/2 cup powdered sugar

For the Coffee Layer:

- 1 cup strong brewed coffee or espresso, cooled to room temperature
- 2 tablespoons coffee liqueur (optional, such as Kahlúa or Tia Maria)

For the Ladyfingers:

- 20-24 ladyfingers (Savoyard)

- **Instructions:**

- 1 teaspoon vanilla extract

- 1 tablespoon unsweetened cocoa powder (for dusting)

1. **Prepare the Cream Layer:**
   o In a mixing bowl, combine the cold heavy cream, mascarpone cheese, powdered sugar, and vanilla extract. Using an electric mixer, beat the mixture on medium-high speed until soft peaks form. Be careful not to overbeat, or the mixture may become grainy. Set aside.

2. **Prepare the Coffee Mixture:**
   o In a shallow dish, combine the cooled coffee or espresso with the coffee liqueur (if using). Stir to mix well.

3. **Dip the Ladyfingers:**
   o Quickly dip each ladyfinger into the coffee mixture, ensuring both sides are moistened but not soaked (they should still hold their shape). Arrange a layer of dipped ladyfingers in the bottom of an 8x8-inch baking dish or a similar-sized dish.

4. **Add the Cream Layer:**
   o Spread half of the mascarpone cream mixture evenly over the layer of ladyfingers in the dish.

5. **Repeat the Layers:**
   o Dip the remaining ladyfingers in the coffee mixture and arrange them on top of the cream layer. Spread the remaining mascarpone cream over the second layer of ladyfingers, smoothing the top with a spatula.

6. **Chill the Tiramisu:**
   o Cover the dish with plastic wrap and refrigerate for at least 4 hours or overnight to allow the flavors to meld and the dessert to set.

7. **Dust with Cocoa Powder:**
   o Just before serving, dust the top of the tiramisu with unsweetened cocoa powder using a fine mesh sieve.

Day 29

Breakfast: Pumpkin Spice Smoothie

Ingredients:

- 1/2 cup pumpkin puree (canned or homemade)

- 1 ripe banana (preferably frozen for a creamier texture)

- 1/2 cup Greek yogurt (or dairy-free yogurt alternative)
- 1 cup almond milk (or your preferred milk)
- 1 tablespoon maple syrup or honey (adjust to taste)
- 1 teaspoon pumpkin pie spice (or a blend of ground cinnamon, nutmeg, ginger, and cloves)

Optional Toppings:

- Whipped cream or coconut whipped cream
- A sprinkle of cinnamon

- 1/2 teaspoon vanilla extract
- A handful of ice cubes (optional, for a thicker smoothie)
- 1 tablespoon chia seeds or flaxseeds (optional, for added nutrition)

- A drizzle of honey or maple syrup
- A few pumpkin seeds or granola for added crunch

Instructions:

1. **Prepare the Ingredients:**
   - If your banana is not already frozen, slice it and freeze it for a few hours for a creamier smoothie.
2. **Blend the Smoothie:**
   - In a blender, combine the pumpkin puree, frozen banana, Greek yogurt, almond milk, maple syrup or honey, pumpkin pie spice, vanilla extract, and ice cubes (if using).
3. **Add Optional Nutrients:**
   - Add chia seeds or flaxseeds to the blender for added fiber and omega-3 fatty acids.

4. **Blend Until Smooth:**
   - Blend on high speed until all ingredients are fully combined and the smoothie is smooth and creamy. If the smoothie is too thick, add a bit more almond milk to reach your desired consistency.
5. **Serve the Smoothie:**
   - Pour the pumpkin spice smoothie into a glass.
6. **Add Optional Toppings:**
   - Top with whipped cream, a sprinkle of cinnamon, a drizzle of honey or maple syrup, and a few pumpkin seeds or granola for added texture and flavor, if desired.

Lunch: Spicy Chicken Lettuce Wraps

Ingredients:

For the Spicy Chicken Filling:

- 1 pound ground chicken
- 1 tablespoon olive oil
- 1/2 red onion, finely chopped
- 2 cloves garlic, minced
- 1 tablespoon fresh ginger, minced
- 1/2 red bell pepper, finely diced
- 2 tablespoons soy sauce or tamari (for a gluten-free option)

- 1 tablespoon hoisin sauce
- 1 tablespoon Sriracha or your preferred hot sauce (adjust to taste)
- 1 tablespoon rice vinegar
- 1 teaspoon sesame oil
- 1/4 teaspoon red pepper flakes (optional, for added heat)
- Salt and pepper to taste

For the Lettuce Wraps:

- 1 head of butter lettuce or iceberg lettuce, leaves separated and washed
- 1/2 cup shredded carrots
- 1/2 cup cucumber, julienned
- 1/4 cup fresh cilantro, chopped

- 1/4 cup green onions, sliced
- 1/4 cup chopped peanuts or cashews (optional, for garnish)
- Lime wedges (optional, for serving)

Instructions:

1. **Prepare the Chicken Filling:**
   - In a large skillet, heat the olive oil over medium heat. Add the chopped red onion, minced garlic, and minced ginger, and sauté for 2-3 minutes, or until the onion is soft and fragrant.
2. **Cook the Ground Chicken:**
   - Add the ground chicken to the skillet and cook, breaking it up with a spoon, for about 5-7 minutes, or until the chicken is fully cooked and no longer pink.
3. **Add the Vegetables and Sauce:**
   - Stir in the diced red bell pepper and cook for an additional 2-3 minutes until the bell pepper is tender. Add the soy sauce or tamari, hoisin sauce, Sriracha, rice vinegar, sesame oil, red pepper flakes (if using), salt, and pepper. Stir well to combine and cook for another 2-3 minutes, allowing the flavors to meld together.
4. **Prepare the Lettuce Wraps:**
   - Arrange the lettuce leaves on a serving platter. Spoon a generous amount of the spicy chicken filling into the center of each lettuce leaf.
5. **Add Toppings:**
   - Top the chicken filling with shredded carrots, julienned cucumber, chopped cilantro, and sliced green onions. Sprinkle with chopped peanuts or cashews for added crunch, if desired.

Dinner: Lemon Garlic Shrimp with Asparagus

Ingredients:

For the Shrimp and Asparagus:

- 1-pound large shrimp, peeled and deveined
- 1 bunch asparagus, trimmed and cut into 2-inch pieces
- 3 tablespoons olive oil, divided
- 4 cloves garlic, minced

- 1/4 teaspoon red pepper flakes (optional, for added heat)
- 1 lemon, zested and juiced
- Salt and pepper to taste
- 2 tablespoons fresh parsley, chopped (optional, for garnish)

Instructions:

1. **Prepare the Ingredients:**
   - Rinse the shrimp under cold water and pat dry with paper towels. Trim the asparagus and cut it into 2-inch pieces.
2. **Cook the Asparagus:**
   - In a large skillet, heat 1 tablespoon of olive oil over medium heat. Add the asparagus pieces and season with salt and pepper. Sauté for 3-4 minutes, or until the asparagus is tender-crisp. Remove the asparagus from the skillet and set aside.
3. **Cook the Shrimp:**

o   In the same skillet, add the remaining 2 tablespoons of olive oil and heat over medium heat. Add the minced garlic and red pepper flakes (if using) and sauté for about 1 minute, or until fragrant.

4. **Add the Shrimp to the Skillet:**
    o   Add the shrimp to the skillet in a single layer. Cook for 2-3 minutes on each side, or until the shrimp are pink and opaque. Be careful not to overcook the shrimp.

5. **Add Lemon Juice and Zest:**
    o   Add the lemon zest and lemon juice to the skillet with the shrimp. Stir to coat the shrimp evenly with the lemon and garlic sauce. Return the cooked asparagus to the skillet and toss to combine.

6. **Season and Garnish:**
    o   Season with additional salt and pepper to taste. Remove from heat and garnish with chopped fresh parsley, if desired.

7. **Serve the Dish:**
    o   Serve the lemon garlic shrimp with asparagus hot, with extra lemon wedges on the side, if desired.

Snack: Whole Grain Crackers with Hummus

Ingredients:

- 1/2 cup hummus (store-bought or homemade)
- 1 cup whole grain crackers (choose low-sodium options for a healthier snack)

Optional Toppings:

- A sprinkle of paprika or cayenne pepper (for added flavor and heat)
- A drizzle of olive oil
- A few chopped fresh herbs, such as parsley or cilantro
- Sliced cucumber, cherry tomatoes, or bell peppers for added crunch

Instructions:

1. **Prepare the Snack:**
    o   Place the whole grain crackers on a serving plate.

2. **Serve with Hummus:**
    o   Scoop the hummus into a small bowl and place it alongside the crackers.

3. **Add Optional Toppings:**
    o   Sprinkle the hummus with paprika or cayenne pepper, drizzle with olive oil, and garnish with fresh herbs if desired.

4. **Add Fresh Vegetables (Optional):**
    o   Serve with additional sliced cucumber, cherry tomatoes, or bell peppers for a fresh, crunchy addition.

Dessert: Strawberry Rhubarb Crisp

Ingredients:

For the Filling:

- 2 cups fresh strawberries, hulled and sliced
- 2 cups fresh rhubarb, sliced (about 1/2-inch thick)
- 1/2 cup granulated sugar
- 1 tablespoon cornstarch
- 1 tablespoon fresh lemon juice
- 1 teaspoon vanilla extract

For the Topping:

- 1 cup rolled oats
- 1/2 cup all-purpose flour (or almond flour for a gluten-free option)
- 1/2 cup brown sugar
- 1/2 teaspoon ground cinnamon
- 1/4 teaspoon salt
- 1/2 cup unsalted butter, melted (or coconut oil for a dairy-free option)

Instructions:

1. **Preheat the Oven:**
   - Preheat your oven to 350°F (175°C). Grease an 8x8-inch baking dish with butter or cooking spray.
2. **Prepare the Filling:**
   - In a large mixing bowl, combine the sliced strawberries, sliced rhubarb, granulated sugar, cornstarch, lemon juice, and vanilla extract. Toss gently to coat the fruit evenly with the sugar and cornstarch. Pour the fruit mixture into the prepared baking dish and spread it out evenly.
3. **Prepare the Topping:**
   - In a separate bowl, mix together the rolled oats, flour, brown sugar, ground cinnamon, and salt. Pour in the melted butter (or coconut oil) and stir until the mixture forms a crumbly texture.
4. **Assemble the Crisp:**
   - Sprinkle the oat topping evenly over the fruit mixture in the baking dish, covering the fruit completely.
5. **Bake the Crisp:**
   - Bake in the preheated oven for 35-40 minutes, or until the topping is golden brown and the fruit filling is bubbly.
6. **Cool and Serve:**
   - Remove the crisp from the oven and let it cool for about 10-15 minutes to allow the filling to set.

Day 30

Breakfast: Sweet Potato and Avocado Breakfast Bowl

Ingredients:

- 1 medium sweet potato, peeled and diced
- 1 tablespoon olive oil
- Salt and pepper to taste
- 1/2 teaspoon smoked paprika (optional)
- 1/2 teaspoon garlic powder (optional)
- 1 ripe avocado, sliced or diced
- 2 large eggs
- 1/2 cup cherry tomatoes, halved
- 1/4 cup black beans, rinsed and drained (optional)

- 1 tablespoon fresh cilantro or parsley, chopped (optional, for garnish)

Instructions:

1. **Roast the Sweet Potatoes:**
   - Preheat your oven to 400°F (200°C). Toss the diced sweet potatoes with olive oil, salt, pepper, smoked paprika, and garlic powder (if using) in a mixing bowl until evenly coated.
   - Spread the sweet potatoes in a single layer on a baking sheet. Roast in the preheated oven for 20-25 minutes, or until the sweet potatoes are tender and slightly crispy, tossing halfway through for even cooking.
2. **Prepare the Eggs:**
   - While the sweet potatoes are roasting, prepare the eggs. You can poach, fry,

- Hot sauce or salsa (optional, for serving)

or scramble the eggs, depending on your preference. Cook until the whites are set, and the yolks are cooked to your desired level of doneness.

3. **Assemble the Breakfast Bowl:**
   - Divide the roasted sweet potatoes between two bowls. Top each bowl with sliced or diced avocado, halved cherry tomatoes, black beans (if using), and the cooked eggs.
4. **Add Optional Garnishes:**
   - Garnish with chopped fresh cilantro or parsley for a burst of color and flavor. Drizzle with hot sauce or salsa, if desired, for added heat and flavor.

Lunch: Chicken Waldorf Salad

Ingredients:

- 2 cups cooked chicken breast, diced or shredded (about 2-3 chicken breasts)
- 1/2 cup celery, finely chopped
- 1/2 cup apple, diced (such as Granny Smith or Honeycrisp)
- 1/2 cup red grapes, halved
- 1/4 cup walnuts, chopped (or pecans)
- 1/4 cup Greek yogurt (or mayonnaise for a richer flavor)

- 1 tablespoon lemon juice
- 1 tablespoon honey or maple syrup (optional, for added sweetness)
- Salt and pepper to taste
- 4 large lettuce leaves (such as Romaine or Bibb lettuce), for serving
- 1/4 cup fresh parsley, chopped (optional, for garnish)

Instructions:

1. **Prepare the Salad Ingredients:**
   - In a large mixing bowl, combine the diced or shredded chicken breast, chopped celery, diced apple, halved grapes, and chopped walnuts.
2. **Make the Dressing:**
   - In a small bowl, whisk together the Greek yogurt, lemon juice, honey or maple syrup (if using), salt, and pepper until smooth and well combined.
3. **Combine Salad and Dressing:**
   - Pour the dressing over the salad ingredients and toss gently to coat everything evenly. Adjust the seasoning with additional salt and pepper to taste.
4. **Chill the Salad (Optional):**
   - For best flavor, cover the bowl with plastic wrap and refrigerate the salad for at least 30 minutes to allow the flavors to meld together.
5. **Serve the Salad:**
   - Place a large lettuce leaf on each serving plate and spoon a generous

portion of the Chicken Waldorf Salad onto each leaf. Alternatively, serve the salad over a bed of mixed greens.

6. **Garnish and Enjoy:**
   o Garnish with fresh parsley, if desired, for added color and flavor.

Dinner: Stuffed Portobello Mushrooms

Ingredients:

- 4 large Portobello mushrooms, stems removed, and gills scraped out
- 2 tablespoons olive oil, divided
- Salt and pepper to taste
- 1/2 cup onion, finely chopped
- 2 cloves garlic, minced
- 1/2 cup bell pepper, finely diced (red or yellow for color)
- 1 cup spinach, chopped
- 1/2 cup cherry tomatoes, quartered
- 1/4 cup breadcrumbs (or gluten-free breadcrumbs)
- 1/4 cup Parmesan cheese, grated (optional)
- 1/2 cup mozzarella cheese, shredded (or dairy-free cheese)
- 1 tablespoon fresh parsley, chopped (optional, for garnish)

Instructions:

1. **Preheat the Oven:**
   o Preheat your oven to 375°F (190°C). Line a baking sheet with parchment paper or lightly grease it with olive oil.
2. **Prepare the Mushrooms:**
   o Brush the Portobello mushrooms with 1 tablespoon of olive oil on both sides and season with salt and pepper. Place them on the prepared baking sheet, gill side up.
3. **Bake the Mushrooms:**
   o Bake the mushrooms in the preheated oven for about 10 minutes to soften them slightly. Remove from the oven and set aside to cool slightly while preparing the filling.
4. **Prepare the Filling:**
   o In a skillet, heat the remaining 1 tablespoon of olive oil over medium heat. Add the chopped onion and sauté for 3-4 minutes, or until softened. Add the minced garlic and bell pepper and cook for another 2-3 minutes, until the vegetables are tender.
5. **Add Spinach and Tomatoes:**
   o Stir in the chopped spinach and cook until wilted, about 1-2 minutes. Add the quartered cherry tomatoes and cook for another 1 minute. Remove the skillet from heat.
6. **Mix the Filling:**
   o Add the breadcrumbs and grated Parmesan cheese (if using) to the vegetable mixture in the skillet. Stir to combine and season with salt and pepper to taste.
7. **Stuff the Mushrooms:**
   o Spoon the filling evenly into each of the pre-baked Portobello mushroom caps. Top each stuffed mushroom with shredded mozzarella cheese.
8. **Bake the Stuffed Mushrooms:**
   o Return the stuffed mushrooms to the oven and bake for an additional 15-20 minutes, or until the cheese is melted and bubbly, and the mushrooms are tender.
9. **Serve the Dish:**
   o Remove the mushrooms from the oven and let them cool slightly before serving.
10. **Garnish and Serve:**
    o Garnish with fresh parsley if desired.

Snack: Yogurt with Honey and Nuts

Ingredients:

- 1 cup plain Greek yogurt (or dairy-free yogurt alternative)
- 1-2 tablespoons honey (adjust to taste)
- 1/4 cup mixed nuts (such as almonds, walnuts, and pecans), chopped

Instructions:

1. **Prepare the Yogurt:**
   - Scoop the Greek yogurt into a bowl.
2. **Add Honey and Nuts:**
   - Drizzle the honey over the yogurt. Sprinkle the chopped nuts on top.

- 1/4 teaspoon ground cinnamon (optional, for added flavor)
- Fresh fruit (such as berries or sliced banana, optional)

3. **Add Optional Toppings:**
   - If desired, sprinkle ground cinnamon over the yogurt for added flavor. Add fresh fruit, such as berries or sliced banana, for extra sweetness and texture.

Dessert: Mango Coconut Pudding

Ingredients:

- 1 1/2 cups ripe mango, diced (about 2 medium mangoes)
- 1 cup coconut milk (full-fat or light, depending on your preference)
- 1/4 cup chia seeds

- 2 tablespoons honey or maple syrup (adjust to taste)
- 1 teaspoon vanilla extract
- 1/4 cup shredded coconut (optional, for garnish)
- Fresh mango slices (optional, for garnish)
- Fresh mint leaves (optional, for garnish)

Instructions:

1. **Prepare the Mango Puree:**
   - In a blender or food processor, puree the diced mango until smooth. Reserve a few mango pieces for garnish, if desired.
2. **Mix the Pudding Ingredients:**
   - In a mixing bowl, combine the mango puree, coconut milk, chia seeds, honey or maple syrup, and vanilla extract. Stir well to ensure the chia seeds are evenly distributed throughout the mixture.
3. **Chill the Pudding:**
   - Cover the bowl with plastic wrap and refrigerate for at least 2 hours, or overnight, to allow the chia seeds to absorb the liquid and thicken into a pudding-like consistency.
4. **Stir the Pudding:**
   - After chilling, give the pudding a good stir to ensure its evenly mixed and the chia seeds haven't clumped together.
5. **Serve the Pudding:**
   - Divide the mango coconut pudding into serving bowls or glasses.
6. **Add Optional Garnishes:**
   - Top with shredded coconut, fresh mango slices, and fresh mint leaves for added flavor and presentation, if desired.

4   Part 3: Maintaining Your Diet Post 30 Days

Tips for Continued Success

After successfully completing your 30-day meal plan, it's important to maintain the healthy eating habits you've developed. Here are some practical tips to help you continue thriving on your gallbladder-friendly diet:

1. **Continue to Choose Whole, Unprocessed Foods:**
   - Focus on incorporating whole foods like fruits, vegetables, whole grains, lean proteins, and healthy fats into your daily meals. These foods are rich in essential nutrients and are easier for your body to digest, especially if you're managing your diet post-gallbladder removal.
2. **Keep Portions in Mind:**
   - Eating in moderation is key to maintaining a balanced diet. Keep portion sizes reasonable to avoid overeating, which can stress your digestive system. Practice mindful eating by paying attention to your hunger and fullness cues.
3. **Stay Hydrated:**
   - Drinking plenty of water is crucial for good digestion and overall health. Aim for at least 8 glasses of water a day and consider herbal teas or infused water with fruits for added flavor and hydration benefits.
4. **Incorporate Healthy Fats:**

- o Include healthy fats such as avocados, nuts, seeds, and olive oil in your diet. These facts are essential for absorbing fat-soluble vitamins and promoting overall health. However, be mindful of your fat intake and avoid high fat, fried, or greasy foods that could trigger digestive discomfort.

5. **Plan Your Meals and Snacks:**
   - o Continue planning your meals and snacks to ensure you're eating a balanced diet and avoiding unhealthy options. Having healthy snacks like fruits, nuts, yogurt, or veggie sticks on hand can help you stay on track.
6. **Experiment with New Recipes:**
   - o Keep your meals exciting by experimenting with new recipes that align with your dietary needs. Try different herbs, spices, and cooking methods to add variety and flavor to your dishes.
7. **Listen to Your Body:**
   - o Pay attention to how your body responds to different foods. Everyone's digestion is unique, so take note of any foods that may cause discomfort or symptoms and adjust your diet accordingly.
8. **Stay Active:**
   - o Regular physical activity can aid digestion, boost metabolism, and improve overall well-being. Incorporate moderate exercise such as walking, yoga, or swimming into your routine to complement your healthy eating habits.
9. **Seek Support:**
   - o Surround yourself with supportive friends and family who understand your dietary needs. Consider joining a support group or online community to share experiences, tips, and recipes with others who are also following a similar diet.
10. **Consult a Healthcare Professional:**
    - o If you have specific dietary concerns or continue to experience digestive issues, consult a healthcare professional, such as a dietitian or gastroenterologist, for personalized advice and guidance.

By following these tips, you can continue to maintain a healthy and balanced diet that supports your digestive health and overall well-being. Remember that consistency and mindful choices are key to long-term success. Celebrate your progress and enjoy the journey to a healthier you!

5   Part 4: Resources and References

Glossary of Ingredients

This glossary provides an overview of some key ingredients used throughout this cookbook. Understanding these ingredients can help you make informed choices about your diet and find suitable substitutions if needed.

---

1. **Almond Butter**: A creamy spread made from ground almonds, often used as a healthier alternative to peanut butter. It's rich in healthy fats, fiber, and protein.
2. **Almond Flour**: A gluten-free flour made from finely ground almonds. It's often used in baking as a low-carb alternative to wheat flour.
3. **Avocado**: A nutrient-dense fruit known for its healthy monounsaturated fats, fiber, and vitamins. It adds creaminess and richness to dishes and is beneficial for heart health.
4. **Balsamic Vinegar**: A dark, sweet, and tangy vinegar made from grape must. It's often used in salad dressings, marinades, and sauces to add depth of flavor.
5. **Cauliflower Rice**: Finely chopped cauliflower that resembles rice grains. It's a low-carb, low-calorie substitute for rice, often used in grain-free and gluten-free recipes.

6. **Chia Seeds**: Small black or white seeds that are rich in fiber, omega-3 fatty acids, and antioxidants. They can absorb liquid and form a gel-like consistency, making them a great addition to smoothies, puddings, and baked goods.
7. **Coconut Milk**: A creamy liquid made from grated coconut flesh, commonly used in Southeast Asian and Caribbean cuisines. It adds a rich, tropical flavor to dishes and is available in both full-fat and light versions.
8. **Edamame**: Young, green soybeans that are often steamed or boiled and served as a snack or added to salads and stir-fries. They are high in protein, fiber, and essential vitamins and minerals.
9. **Feta Cheese**: A tangy, crumbly cheese traditionally made from sheep's or goat's milk. It is often used in Mediterranean dishes such as salads, wraps, and baked goods.
10. **Flaxseeds**: Small brown or golden seeds rich in fiber, omega-3 fatty acids, and lignans. They can be ground into a powder and used as an egg substitute in vegan baking or added to smoothies and cereals for added nutrition.
11. **Greek Yogurt**: A thick, creamy yogurt that is strained to remove excess whey, resulting in a higher protein content. It can be used in both savory and sweet dishes as a healthier alternative to sour cream or mayonnaise.
12. **Hummus**: A creamy spread made from blended chickpeas, tahini (sesame seed paste), lemon juice, garlic, and olive oil. It is commonly used as a dip or spread and is a good source of protein, fiber, and healthy fats.
13. **Kale**: A leafy green vegetable that is high in vitamins A, C, and K, as well as fiber and antioxidants. It can be eaten raw in salads or cooked in various dishes.
14. **Nutritional Yeast**: A deactivated yeast with a cheesy, nutty flavor often used in vegan and dairy-free recipes as a cheese substitute. It is rich in B vitamins and provides a savory umami taste to dishes.
15. **Quinoa**: A gluten-free grain-like seed that is high in protein, fiber, and essential amino acids. It cooks quickly and can be used in salads, side dishes, and breakfast bowls.
16. **Rolled Oats**: Whole oats that have been steamed and flattened, commonly used in oatmeal, baking, and as a binder in recipes like veggie burgers. They are a good source of fiber and help lower cholesterol levels.
17. **Tahini**: A paste made from ground sesame seeds, often used in Middle Eastern and Mediterranean cuisine. It adds a rich, nutty flavor to dishes and is a key ingredient in hummus and salad dressings.
18. **Tamari**: A gluten-free soy sauce alternative made from fermented soybeans. It has a rich, savory flavor and is commonly used in Asian cuisine and as a seasoning in various dishes.
19. **Tofu**: A versatile, high-protein food made from coagulated soy milk. It comes in different textures (silken, soft, firm, extra firm) and can be used in a wide range of savory and sweet dishes.
20. **Turmeric**: A bright yellow spice made from the root of the turmeric plant. It has a warm, earthy flavor and is often used in curries, soups, and rice dishes. Turmeric is known for its anti-inflammatory properties and health benefits.
21. **Zoodles**: Noodles made from spiralized zucchini, often used as a low-carb and gluten-free alternative to traditional pasta. They are light, versatile, and can be used in various dishes, including salads and stir-fries.

By familiarizing yourself with these ingredients, you'll be better equipped to prepare the recipes in this cookbook and adapt them to your personal preferences or dietary needs.

Conclusion

Congratulations on completing the 30-day meal plan and taking significant steps toward improving your digestive health and overall well-being! By embracing a gallbladder-friendly diet, you've not only supported your body's ability to digest and absorb nutrients effectively, but you've also cultivated a sustainable approach to eating that nourishes both body and mind.

As you move forward, remember that maintaining a healthy diet is a lifelong journey. Continue to explore new recipes, listen to your body's needs, and stay informed about the best practices for your digestive health. The habits you've built over these past 30 days will serve as a strong foundation for your continued success.

Thank you for choosing this cookbook as your guide. May it continue to inspire you to create delicious, nourishing meals that support your health goals. Here's to a healthier, happier you!

Bon Appétit!